"It is not the strongest of the species that survives, nor the most intelligent. It is the one that is most adaptable to change." - Charles Darwin (attributed)

"You try to plant something in the concrete, y'know what I mean? If it grow, and the rose petal got all kind of scratches and marks, you not gonna say, 'Damn, look at all the scratches and marks on the rose that grew from concrete'; you gonna be like, 'Damn! A rose grew from the concrete?!'" – Tupac Shakur

The

Kitchen Sink Farming

Series

Volume 3: Growing [Edition 1]

Publisher:

Stone Soup Publications

Portland, OR 97239

publisher@KitchenSinkFarming.org

©2012 Jean-Pierre Parent

No part of this book may be reproduced or transmitted in any form or by any means, electronic or mechanical, including photocopying or recording or by any information storage or retrieval systems without prior permission in writing from Stone Soup Publications or Jean-Pierre Parent.

In humble gratitude to the trees that grew to make the paper recycled to make this book. I've tried to use you wisely.

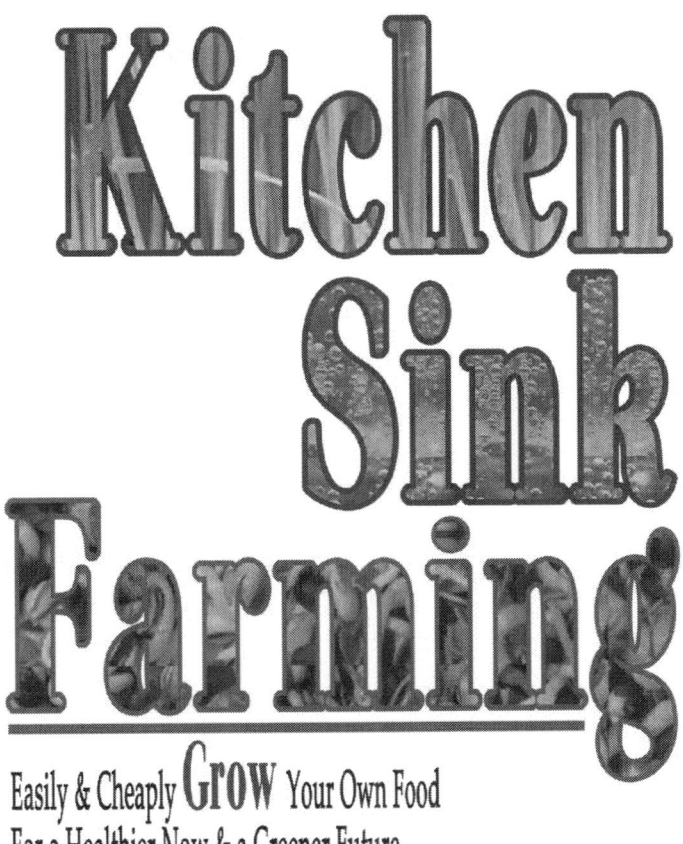

Easily & Cheaply Grow Your Own Food
For a Healthier Now & a Greener Future

Volume 2

in the Kitchen Sink Farming Series

Jean-Pierre Parent

Also by Jean-Pierre Parent:

In the "Kitchen Sink Farming" Series:

- Vol 1: Sprouting
- Vol 2: Fermenting
- Vol 3: Growing
- Vol 4: Homegrown Living Recipes - What to Do with Your Sprouts and Krauts
- The Complete Set: all 4 Volumes

And

Practice Makes... Meditation and Yoga in Everyday Life

JP's blogs

Food: www.KitchenSinkFarming.org

Yoga: www.OmInvasion.org

Contents

The "Why?" 12
Table 1: Effects of Sprouting on Mung Beans 16
A Deeper Reason to Take Control of Our Food: Truly Empty Calories 18
A History of Agri-Tech 19
Burger & a Side of Flies: Genetic Modification of Food .. 20
When Organic Isn't (It's too easy being green) 28
Collapse, the Future of Food 34
Peak Oil Pioneers 36
Easter Island's Last Lumberjack 41
Everyone but the Kitchen Sink: Modernization, McDonald's, and Hyper-Maturation 45
Changing Food Habits - Using the Brain for a Change 50
Transitioning to a Living Diet 54
   Table 2: Seed/Nut Digestibility Chart 55
Growing 58
   Why Grow Grass? 59
   The Benefits of Wheatgrass Grass Juice 61
   How to Grow and Enjoy Grasses 68
   Dirt 69
   Dealing with dirt in an apartment 70
   Soilless Media 73
   Containers 76
   Light 77
   Fertilization - Feed Your Soil, Not Your Plants 80
   H, P, and That Sneaky Little O: Hydrogen Peroxide 83

How to Juice Grass 87

Micro-Lettuces, Shoots and Greens 88

Choosing your plants.. 89

Start a new batch when your current crop is a week in, and you'll have micro-lettuce salads all year round. 91

Shoots 91

Sunflower Lettuce 92

Container Gardening.. 94

Outdoor Growing 94

Light... 95

Choosing Crops 100

Indoor Growing 102

Self-Watering Containers 102

Simple Self-Watering Devices: "the spike" and "the holey bottle" 103

The Watering Spike 103

The Self-Watering Bucket 104

The Self-Watering Garden 107

Fertilizing... 108

Hooked on 'Ponics: Hydroponic and Aeroponic Gardening 109

The Plans: Hydroponics... 112

Small-Scale Set-Up 115

Large-Scale Hydro Set-up 120

The Growing Wall.. 126

Barrel and Drum Gardening.. 136

DIY Aeroponics 140

The Aero-Tote	140
Composting and Worm-iculture	148
DIY Tumbling Composter	155
Appendix A - Plant Nutritional Deficiencies	188
Recommended Reading	193
Resources:	195
Index	173

Preface

This book is the result of a serious personality flaw.

Somehow, from a very early age, I've rarely been satisfied with anything. Or, more accurately, I'm only satisfied with perfection, that acutely rare and delicate moment when the stars align; the air is just so, filling the lungs with sweet fortitude and the project before you sparkles with temporal rightness...

This eternal dissatisfaction with the lack of perfection pervades every aspect of my life: my athleticism, health, relationships, even conversations. I practiced them beforehand, and I think about them afterwards, re-working them in my mind until my responses are the most thoughtful, compassionate, wise, and considerate statements possible. When I was a little kid playing with my Atari, I probably hit the reset button on the console more often than the one on the controller, starting the game over and over if I did something that wasn't *quite* right, so that I could have a chance to do it again, and this time, perfectly. At the time, I think I expected all of life could be like that.

But I think I really hit my "always-satisfied-with-the-best" stride with food. If I was eating something (and that happened quite often in those days), I would wonder "what's the best possible form of this food?" So I cut out junk food and soda (I think I was nine at this time), after experiencing how I felt after eating a fast food hamburger before a soccer game. Didn't make that mistake again. I soon came to learn about vegetarian, then vegan, then organic, then raw food. The quest didn't stop there though, because of the widely varying ideas of raw vs. living food, organic standards, and genetic modification of food. Recently, the world's largest chain of natural food grocery stores was caught selling frozen vegetables as organic that were actually grown in China with little respect for chemical-free farming, and the "independent" organic certifiers that permitted the labeling are owned by the store (more on pg 30). So it's a constant question about who's trustworthy, and "how long will they be?" (See chapter "Truly Empty Calories", subchapter *"When Organic Isn't (It's Too Easy Being Green)"* for more on this particular paranoia).

And then there is the immeasurable question of taste. All this wholesome, nutritious food (like the bland and boring natural choices when I was a kid and 90% of them today) might be good for the body but unless it can create sublime waves of closed-eye, tilted-headed moaning pleasure, it does little for the soul. And therefore leaves something to be desired. Incomplete. Imperfect.

These days, my slightly mellowed aspirations for perfection have made me an experimenter, a scientist, a chef, a do-it-yourself-er. Before sitting down to write this (at a desk that I built so I could be the perfect height, with a pillow that I cut from the perfect density of memory foam mattress, on which I am sitting in a yoga position called siddhasana, or perfect pose) I noticed that some pumpkin seeds I sprouted and put in my dehydrator for a crunchy snack were sticking together. Makes sense, if you've ever lobotomized a pumpkin for a jack-o-lantern, scooping out its slimy stuck-together seeds. I thought that natural cohesion might be a good start to a flatbread, maybe mixed with super-sticky flax. So, did I make *a* pumpkinseed-flax flatbread? No... I made about 2 dozen. Equal parts flax and pumpkin. Double one, and double the other. Each one of those split in thirds, one part put on the counter to ferment, one in the oven at a low temp, and the rest in the dehydrator at a lower temp.

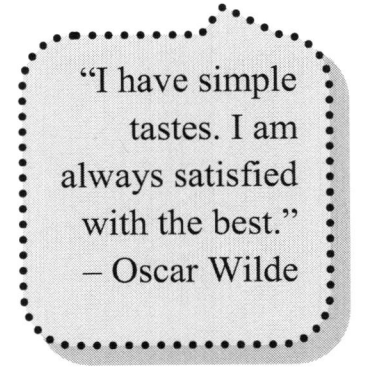

> "I have simple tastes. I am always satisfied with the best."
> – Oscar Wilde

Each of *those* split in half again, dry or with some oil. One in each category blended with some sprouted spelt, to see if they'd be better a little cake-ier. All labeled and catalogued. You get the idea.

Some may think that this level precision is boring, rigid, anal-retentive, or obsessive, and I might agree if it was focused on a less important subject. But I think nourishment is just too important to be satisfied with anything less than utterly thorough knowledge, which until recently we've had to mostly figure by our lonesomes. I think that this mindset is an integral part of being able to draw the measure of life's awesomeness and maybe the best way to experience the most happiness, fun, health, contentedness, and eventual freedom, because I will *know* what the best choice is for me today. With certainty. That's the goal, anyways. And then I'm happy, because the mundane turns into magic when it's dove into with attentive and receptive enthusiasm.

This book is the result of my decades-long experiment that asks the question: what's the best food possible, to fuel the best life possible? I think I've found glimmers of the answer, and I'm so pleased to be able share them with you.

This is what led me to eating whole, organic, living foods: wanting to get as much out of my food as possible. Your reasons might be totally different. Starting with pure ingredients is a life-saver for someone with food allergies – the only way to take control of what goes into your body. Even someone lactose intolerant can enjoy the bowel-healing properties of milk (as raw kefir,), butter (as ghee), or cheeses of many kinds (all in Kitchen Sink Farming Volume 2: Fermenting). Cancer patients find remission through fermented foods. The environmental benefits of enough home growers and sprouters will have a major global impact. A network of neighbors that each specialize in a different product could build community like nothing else – focused around the most primal and fundamental cement of society. And as I'll mention time and again, it's also the cheapest way to eat what is possibly the very best food in the world.

The "Why?"

The world's best foods aren't available in stores. You can't get them from the home shopping network, either. It's a good thing, too, because then people would buy them and miss out on the particular satisfaction of eating something they grew themselves, acutely aware of the life cycle of and organic rhythms of nature in their current mouthful. It's also a good thing because they're really cheap and nearly really easy to make, and once you try it, it'd be laughable to pay someone else to do it. This book is based on the firm fact that anyone, anywhere, at any time, can be enjoying a bounty of fresh, living, incredibly nutritious food with very little work and expense.

Once you've enjoyed a delicious and vibrant lunch made from sprouted seeds, grains, or nuts bursting with taste and life, you won't need any convincing. You'll know by that point how easy, cheap, and fun it is to grow sweet strawberries, succulent micro greens, and juicy tomatoes with shocking depth of flavor in your seventh-story apartment kitchen, washing them down with home-brewed, wild-yeasted ginger ale or sparkling kombucha tea. In the meantime, though, before you figure all that out for yourself, it's supportive to know exactly why you're doing what you're doing. Maybe you're interested in increasing the amount of fresh, organic food you're eating (and

> "A great revolution in just one single individual will help achieve a *change* in the destiny of a society and, further, will enable a *change* in in the destiny of humankind."
> *Daisaku Ikeda*

there's no fresher food than something grown 5 feet away from your table and "picked" when you take your first chew!) and dramatically improving your health, energy, and immune system. Maybe you want to save money on groceries or have less of an impact on the earth, casting a vote against industrialized, destructive modern farming methods. Or maybe girls (and guys) just wanna have fun in the kitchen. Whatever your reason, learning about the myriad benefits of sprouting, indoor gardening, and fermenting at home will only encourage and inspire. And it just might make you able to explain to your mom why the dinner peas have leaves.

Nutrients and enzymes don't take kindly to cooking, canning, or sitting on shelves. Even fresh, organic produce loses valuable benefits every hour it's wilting away under the grocery store lights. In Los Angeles, it's hard to walk a few blocks and not pass a Whole Foods or organic restaurant. But even there, in the city with perhaps the greatest access to all things health, sprouted peanut butter, Kamut grass juice (wheat's superior ancestor), unpasteurized sauerkraut, enzymatically-active hot soups, and raw goat milk kefir are not for sale or else have to be painstakingly and expensively tracked down, even though these examples of the most healthful versions of common foods require very little knowledge, no expensive equipment, and less than a minute a day to make. When I was learning the things in this book, even though my efforts usually required a lot of trial and error, I kept coming back to the same eureka feeling: "It *can't* be this easy." But it is. A short and hopefully fun learning adventure will have you eating better than ever before, saving money, and feeling amazing. Maybe one day your local Piggly Wiggly will have a nut butter cafe, where they'll grind the freshly sprouted nuts of your choice, which you can spread on the apple a polite and well-groomed apron-clad deli worker just picked in front of you. If and when we get there through the slow and painstaking process of transforming consumer opinion and convincing the huge conglomerates that it's cost-effective to service us in this way, they'll surely charge an arm and a snout for it. No. The only way to eat living, vital, delicious food is to grow and prepare it yourself.

Nature is a hard-working and dedicated employee. Hire her to work for you and then sit back and relax. Nobody fertilizes or irrigates the forest. It's a complete system that does these things on its own. Make a "food forest" in your apartment, home, or patio, and your main effort is to pick the food. You put in some effort at the very beginning, but once the system is established, you work a lot less. You could call kitchen sink farming "lazy agriculture", because you're working *with* nature, and not against it. You're using the laws of nature, forces that apply equally on a rainforest floor, a Brooklyn backyard, or a Tokyo high-rise to grow your lunch. Sprouting, fermenting, and growing your own food are plain and simple the best foods you can get. They're the least amount of energy to digest, the most nutrition, the least impact on the environment, resources, and humanity for the longest, most disease and discomfort-free life. And wouldn't you know it: it's the cheapest and easiest way to create food, too. Anyone in the world can apply at least one principal in this

> **Nerd Corner!**
>
> Sprouting seeds increases their nutrient availability by 50-2000%, with an average of about 500%. See table on pages 14-15 to see the effects on specific nutrients after sprouting mung beans (not the most common spout, but possibly the most fun to say).

book, and the more you work into your own everyday life, the better off that life will be for it.

Sprouting: Why Mess with a Perfectly Good Seed?

1) Sprouting activates enzymes.

Sprouts have an average of 7 times the enzymes needed to digest them, enzymes that can go to work digesting other foods, repairing and regenerating the body. See page 62 for more on enzymes.

> "Intelligence is the ability to adapt to change."
> Stephen Hawking

2) Sprouting Increases Nutrition

Sprouted seeds supply nutrients in a predigested form – food is broken down into its simplest and easiest-to-digest components. During sprouting, much of the starch is broken down into simple sugars such as glucose and sucrose by the action of the enzyme 'amylase'. Proteins are converted into amino acids and amides. Fats and oils are converted into more simple fatty acids by the enzyme lipase. Sprouts are also high in fiber, so that along with their water helps digestion even more.

3) Sprouting removes "Enzyme Inhibitors"

Enzyme Inhibitors keep seeds from sprouting at the wrong time, and keep nutrients locked up. Sprouting seeds makes them easier to digest and more nutritious for this reason as well, and actually makes everything you eat before and after more nutritious too. (see pg 62 for more)

Table 1: Effects of Sprouting on Mung Beans

First two columns of chart reprinted from Critical Reviews in Food Science and Nutrition, 1989; 28(5):401-37. "Nutritional improvement of cereals by sprouting", Chavan JK, Kadam SS., Department of Biochemistry, Mahatma Phule Agricultural University, Rahuri, India.

Protein	Increases 30%	The increase in protein availability is an indicator of the overall enhancement of nutritional value of a sprouted seed.
Carbohydrates	Decreases 15%	The simultaneous reduction in carbohydrate and caloric content indicates that many carbohydrate molecules are broken down during sprouting to allow absorption of atmospheric nitrogen to reform it into amino acids. The resulting protein is the most easily digestible of all proteins.
Calcium	Increases 30%	
Potassium	Increases 80%	
Sodium	Increases 690%	The skyrocketing sodium content is a good indication that foods are much more easily

		digestible in the sprouted form, as sodium is essential to the digestive process, particularly in the intestines, and also to the elimination of carbon dioxide. The building blocks of both nutrition and digestibility peak simultaneously.
Iron	Increases 40%	
Vitamin A	Increases 285%	
Vitamin B1 (Thiamine)	Increases 208%	
Vitamin B2 (Riboflavin)	Increases 515%	
Vitamin B3 (Niacin)	Increases 256%	
Vitamin C	Infinite Increase	Dry seeds don't show a measurable amount of Vitamin C, but it skyrockets when they're sprouted. Vitamin C is important in the metabolization of proteins, which also increase in sprouted seeds.

A Deeper Reason to Take Control of Our Food: Truly Empty Calories

Food that's not organically grown by traditional, natural methods (paradoxically called "conventionally-grown"), is fairly devoid of nutrients. Large-scale commercial farmers discovered in the 1940's that three nutrients are required to grow and produce normal-looking crops: nitrogen, phosphorous, and potassium, or NPK, but plants, like us, require over 100 minerals to be at their best, and if it's not in the soil, it's not on your plate. Plants grown "conventionally" don't have the nutrients they need to develop healthy immune systems, requiring farmers to spray them down with a heavy coat of pesticides, herbicides, and fungicides. When we eat the fruit and vegetables that comes off of nutrient-deficient, chemical pesticide-laden plants, we suffer in two ways: very little nutrition and a dose of cancer-causing chemicals. When I'm travelling and can't get organic produce, I feel as if I'm eating photographs of food. The apples look like apples, they're red and round, but they're tasteless and my body feels a lifeless chunk of food in my belly as if I've been chewing on paper. My body is waiting for the flood of nourished happiness that it's used to, but doesn't come.

It gets worse. Turns out this disconnect is the well-planned stratagem of big business, who can almost always be counted on to put profits before people. Consumers are starting to become aware of a decades-old curtain of misinformation and propaganda drawn between grocery store shoppers and the contents of their carts by massive agribusiness and their bigger, cheaper, faster business model. But it wasn't always this way.

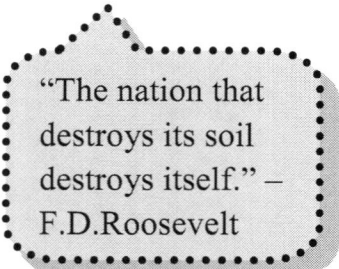
"The nation that destroys its soil destroys itself." – F.D.Roosevelt

A History of Agri-Tech

Before World War II, people farmed the way they always have: fertilizing their fields with nutrient-dense organic matter or growing where rivers overflow and deposit the year's worth of mineral-rich silt. They rotated crops so that plants that take certain nutrients from the soil are supported by a season of plants that put those nutrients back. They relied on the strength of the crops' own immunity to fight off pests. Rainbows glittered over every dew-speckled family-farmed field of organic heirloom veggies… Ok, not really, but food *was* more nutritious and less carcinogenic.

> "Humanity consumed 120% of the earth's sustainable resource capacity in 1999" - National Academy of Sciences, June

World War II inspired many advances in industrial science, from napalm and synthetic rubber to the atomic bomb. When it was over, huge stocks of nitrates from ammunition building, organophosphates for making nerve gas, and other chemicals had accumulated. Nitrates contain nitrogen, one component of the NPK triad, and an enterprising chemical company re-labeled them "fertilizer". Nerve agents like mustard gas, shown to block communication between the brain and organs in both humans and insects alike, were called "pesticides", and both of these were sold to post-war farms. These chemicals, with only slight variations are still used today, and over 1.5 million pounds of organophosphates are sprayed every year on California farms alone.

The huge demand placed on modern farmers to feed more and more people on less and less space is creating an unparalleled desperation. In an attempt to keep up with demand, farmers have fired nature and are courting the promise of a dangerous and only partially-understood technology.

Burger & a Side of Flies: Genetic Modification of Food

Pick a single-ingredient food off the supermarket shelves and you have a 70% chance of grabbing a genetically modified organism, or GMO. This is the volatile and very scary process of splicing a fruit, veggie, or grain's DNA with genes from another organism, always part bacteria, often animal and sometimes even insect, human, or virus. Choose something with corn (or a derivative like corn syrup, dextrose, baking powder, caramel and caramel coloring, mono and diglicerides, modified food starch, vegetable anything: broth, oil, protein, shortening, and the many other ways industrious food scientists have found to pump the most heavily-subsidized and therefore most commonly-grown crop in the US into our diets) or a food with more than a few ingredients and unless it's organic or specifically labeled "non-GMO" your chances go up to around 100%. The ancient process of plant breeding is this: put two plants with traits you like next to each other and hope they'll cross-pollinate and the next generation will be an even better plant.

This wasn't precise or fast enough for modern agri-business. GMO was born out of the desire to achieve total dominion over crops, under the guise of lowering costs and increasing yields. But as with the attempt to control most things in nature, the outcome was not the expected one. Genetic modification has actually cost agriculture more, after recalls on untamable seeds, the inability of GM plants to access nutrients in the soil, puzzlingly lower yields in drought conditions and increased needs for more powerful pesticides with the consequence of mutant super-weeds. None of these issues have impeded cell-invasive technology's expansion, however, as the planting of BT crops went from zero acres in 1988 to 3.7 million in 1996 to 100 million in 2003. Most of the financial burden has fallen not on the slick-talking companies, however, but on the farmers who were taken in by their glimmering promises. It becomes a deadly gamble when, like between 2001 and 2005, 32,000 Indian farmers committed suicide underneath the avalanche of debt an Indian subsidiary of the Monsanto Corporation pawned off onto them when their GM cotton fields were ravaged by a disease that affected only GM plants. Ironically, at least one of the farmers killed himself, at 25 years old, by drinking a liter of pesticide.

Monsanto is one of the companies that is single-handedly destroying the traditional methods of farming in favor of a near-fascist domination of farmers and the very DNA of the seeds they plant, and along with it the worlds' food supply. Monsanto, whose first success was Agent Orange, the forest defoliant used in the Vietnam are and has since been found guilty in Federal courts of falsifying their earnings statements (Foreign Corrupt Practices Act (15 U.S.C. § 78dd-1)), bribing government officials around the globe (15 U.S.C § 78m(b)(2) & (5)), knowingly polluting the small town of Anniston, Alabama, with dangerous levels of polychlorinated biphenyls (PCBs) resulting in over 3.500 cases of cancer and other degenerative diseases, mislabeling pesticides to minimize their dangers (*Monsanto guilty of chemical poisoning in France,* Reuters Feb 13, 2012) and countless other crimes against humankind and nature. In the year 2000, it was estimated that 10 new people everyday are diagnosed with cancer due to exposure to dioxin produced by Monsanto (US Environmental Protection Agency's (EPA) draft reassessment on dioxin) and as of this writing, Monsanto is being taken to court by a group of Argentinean tobacco farmers who say that the biotech giant knowingly poisoned them with herbicides and pesticides and subsequently caused "devastating birth defects" in their children.

But the *really* scary part of this whole mess is that these "franken-foods" reproduce in unexpected and uncontrollable ways. Bizarre monstrosities of barely recognizable plants discovered in fields. 1000-generational heirloom corn farms contaminated by invading mutant DNA. Monsanto's BT corn, cotton, and soy are *themselves* registered as pesticides. The process of genetically modifying foods is not only unethical and disgusting, but we're messing with forces we don't understand and the current results are hinting at world-wide epidemics of sci-fi horror film proportions. For example, in 1989 there was an outbreak of a new disease in the US, traced back to a batch of an L-tryptophan food supplement produced with GMO bacteria. Though it contained less than .1% of the highly

> "A molecular study conducted by Mexican, American and Dutch researchers demonstrates the presence of genes from genetically modified organisms (GMO) among the varieties of traditional corn cultivated in the remote regions of Oaxaca State in the southern part of the country, even though the Mexican government has always maintained a moratorium on the use of transgenic seed." - from "GMO Contamination in Mexico's Cradle of Corn" *Le Monde*, December 11 2008

toxic compound, 37 people died that year and 1,500 were left with permanent disabilities.

The Food and Drug Administration declared that it was not gene modification that was at fault but a failure in the purification process. However, the company concerned, Showa Denko, admitted that the low-level purification process had been used without ill effect in non-GM batches. Scientists at Showa Denko blame the GM process for producing traces of a potent new toxin, and this new toxin had never been found in non-GM versions of the product. In May 2008, new findings by the Physicians and Scientists for Responsible Application of Science and Technology (PSRAST) caused them to state "Most importantly, the poison considered most important in the tryptophan was closely similar to tryptophan (a dimer), but never found in natural bacteria. This indicates that disturbed tryptophan metabolism generated the poison. Moreover, the inserted genes were directed at altering the metabolism (so as to increase tryptophan production).

> "Typically, if something is to be considered Generally Recognized as Safe (G.R.A.S.) it needs lots of peer-reviewed published studies and an overwhelming consensus among the scientific community. With GM crops, they had neither." – Jeffrey Smith, author, *Seeds of Deception*

Our conclusion is that the only plausible explanation for the appearance of this poison is disturbances of the natural metabolic processes due to genetic engineering."

This is just one example of the dangers of genetic manipulation. It's easy to imagine that every instance of genetic modification has its own tale, or will. In fact, children have more adverse reactions to GMOs than adults, and it's hard to not picture a future without horrible consequences from freely fucking with nature. The idea hits home even harder when a public official in Japan,

> From news footage of Vice President George Bush Sr. at the Monsanto factory in 1987:
>
> Monsanto Executive: "We have no complaint about the way the USDA is handling it; they're going through an orderly process… Now if we're waiting til September and we don't have our authorization we may say something different!"
>
> Bush: "Call me. We're in the de-reg [de-regulation] business. Maybe we can help."

where GM foods are outlawed stated their plan to "watch US children for the next ten years" before they determine their next course of action, according to the documentary "The Future of Food" (Deborah Koons Garcia, Lily Films, 2004).

Bio-engineered foods don't have, and were never designed, to provide any benefit to the consumer. No attempt has been made to make more nutritious wheat or better-tasting spinach. Instead, the GM industry's only goal is profit (of everyone but the farmer), so the scam has been sold to the American consumer as a way to provide food for the masses of overpopulated future generations. One problem with this logic is that the nearly 1 billion malnourished people (10,000 of which die every day from starvation) don't do so because of a lack of food. Many of these people used to be farmers, but were kicked off their land when their respective governments accepted huge loans from multi-national banks, and subsistence farming wasn't a workable way to pay them back. Forced off their farms and into the slums of industrializing third-world cities, they have gone from being food independent to food-dependant. The calamitous issue of world hunger is not a problem of production; it's a crisis of access, which is strange when one considers that the average piece of food travels 1500 miles from the farm to the supermarket. The other argument with this propaganda is Monsanto's plan to include in all seeds they produce a "terminator gene", a self-destructing abomination that creates a plant with sterile progeny. That means that if you buy a seed from Monsanto and plant it, instead of being able to harvest the seeds from your plants for next year, you will have to buy more seeds. This is clear proof that the biotech industry has no interest in "feeding the world", as their propaganda states. In the same way that GMO seeds have mysteriously found their way into native plant genes (see quote below), the danger of this terminator gene out-crossing into the plants that make up the world's food supply, effectively ending traditional,

> "AG Biotech will find a supporter occupying the White House next year, regardless of which candidate wins the election in November."
> – Monsanto In-House Newsletter, Oct 6 2000, in reference to the multiple White House officials that are also board members of Monsanto.

sustainable farming, must have gone unnoticed by the company's scientists and members of the USDA who both approved the use of the gene and co-own it. No one can be that evil.

But who is responsible if terminator genes cross-contaminate unsuspecting food supplies? By past precedent, it's not the seed company that's to blame but the farmer, and courts have told farmers that by not protecting their fields properly from seeds blowing in (an absolutely ludicrous idea), they have unwittingly signed a contract with the biotech company that's patented that specific invading gene. Is it possible that one day the world's entire food supply will be controlled by the company that brought us PCB's (which are present in the cells of every man, woman, and child on Earth), DDT, bovine growth hormone, and dioxins, and who has bribed government officials to look the other way while illegally dumping 50 tons of mercury into one Alabama river, stating "We cannot afford to lose one dollar of business" in an internal memo (a leaked copy of which is readily available online) when this criminal polluting was exposed?

Monsanto does, however, have most of America's, and soon the world's, farmers completely dependent on them each planting season. And their wrath is swift and brutal against farmers even suspected of saving viable seeds. Even farmers with neighboring fields that have had these manipulated genes carried by the wind into their crops, which then cross into the genes of the new plants, are pressured with debilitating lawsuits to either go out-of-business or sign a contract and enter into the cycle of dependence and perversion.

Not surprisingly, by current FDA regulations, GMO foods

> "We received over 44,000 pages from the FDA's own files and they revealed that the FDA has been lying to the world since 1992, if not before. But they continue to lie, they're still lying, they claim that there's an overwhelming consensus in the scientific community that genetically engineered foods are as safe as their conventionally produced counterparts and they claim that there has been sufficient data to back up this consensus. [Based on the FDA files] both of those claims are blatant lies." Steven Druker, lawyer for the Alliance for Bio-Integrity, who forced the FDA to unclassify its internal files on GMOs.

aren't allowed to be labeled as such.

And back to the history… After WWII, famers began growing just one crop on a field, requiring more and more chemical support as the malnourished plants weakened. In fact, according to the National Resources Defense Council, pesticide use since the 1940's has gone up 10 times, but crop loss due to insects has doubled, and in the meantime the Environmental Protection Agency estimates that there are pesticide residuals in the

> "This [genetic modification of food] is the largest biological experiment humanity has ever entered into." – Dr. Ignacio Chapel, Microbial Biologist, UC Berkeley

tissues of every American. Our current agricultural system now relies on toxic fertilizers to keep the land producing food, as the precious topsoil that took thousands of years to develop is being washed away at an alarming rate. In fact, in the last 50 years, America has lost over 75% of its fertile soil. It takes 200 to 1000 years to create just one inch of topsoil; no modern technology can make it faster than that. Add to that the fact that the world's main food-producing countries like the US, China, India, Australia and Spain have or are about to reach their water resource limits, and you have an unsustainable agricultural system that can't go on this way much longer. Our dependence on chemical agriculture is a slippery slope. Like hard drugs, we need more and more to get the same affects. Something's gotta give, or soon there will be no seeds to sow, no topsoil to sow them in, no water to water them with, and certainly no way to protect them from the very gentlest of bugs. The only way out is for you and me to take responsibility for what we're putting into our bodies by growing it ourselves, not just voting for change but passionately and peacefully dissenting against an untenable system by planting or sprouting a seed and eating it with delight.

There is hope that the US will follow the example of Europe and Japan who, not beholden to the rebates, subsidies and political and collegiate contributions of the biotech industries, have outlawed all GM foods. A federal judge recently invalidated the patent on a gene that is known to cause breast cancer, owned by Myriad Genetics in association with the University of Utah, who charged exorbitant fees to research facilities using the gene to research breast cancer prevention. This ruling casts doubt on the motives of the companies holding gene patents and raises important ethical questions about the ability to patent life.

When Organic Isn't (It's too easy being green)

Obviously, it's better to buy organic food over conventional. It's a vote for the health of your family, your community, and the environment. Unfortunately, just choosing produce with an organic sticker isn't enough. I want to believe the strict and stringent guidelines for organic certification are followed by

> "If we're still dragging our feet in 2015, it really becomes almost impossible for the world to avert a degree of climate change that we simply will not be able to manage", John Holdren, Professor of Environmental Policy, Harvard University, and Director of the White House Office of Science

participating farms with enthusiasm and far-sighted wisdom, but I know too much about the funding the certifiers receive from the corporations whose goal it is to relax the laws for the betterment of their immediate profits. I hear too many stories from friends in the biz who are told to slap an organic sticker on every fifth crate of asparagus they're packing and call it a day. In 2005 in the UK, the wide-spread epidemic of fraudulently labeling meat as organic was a scandal that required a major government crackdown. The USDA, America's main certification agency who both makes the rules and sells organic certification, is heavily funded by Monsanto and other biotech conglomerates. It's companies like these that are fighting for (and paying for) more lenient rules within an increasingly lucrative market.

And it's working: a 2006 amendment created a list of 38 synthetic ingredients allowed in products that can still be called organic. This allowed Anheuser-Busch in 2007 to have its "Wild Hop Lager" certified organic even though it uses hops grown with chemical fertilizers and sprayed with pesticides. Advocacy groups fear that, since almost all organic foods are now sold through high-volume distribution channels like Target and Wal-Mart (the #1 retailer of organics in the US), the laws will change to support the massive producers, and the small farms that pioneered traditional methods of farming will be squeezed out. While they wait for the laws to change, Wal-mart continually pressures their suppliers to cut corners, if not to break laws outright. In 2007, Aurora Organic Dairy, Wal-mart's main supplier of organic dairy products, was found to be in violation of 14 organic regulations and would have lost their certification if it weren't for some unusual leniency on the part of the FDA. The truth is, the organic label can be bought, and is at best a vague indication of standards practiced in fields and facilities. On the other side of the coin, many small farms that operate according to organic guidelines and beyond aren't certified simply because they can't afford to be.

The simple truth is that big business cannot be trusted to do the right thing when millions or billions of dollars are at stake. Advertisers use buzz words like "fresh", "family-owned", "natural", "local" not in an effort to accurately describe, but to sell with little interest in the truth. It's gotten quite out of hand how advertisers can say absolutely anything and we, in our nose-to-the-grindstone haste to feel better, or check "good for us" off of our grocery lists, let ourselves be unthinkingly swayed.

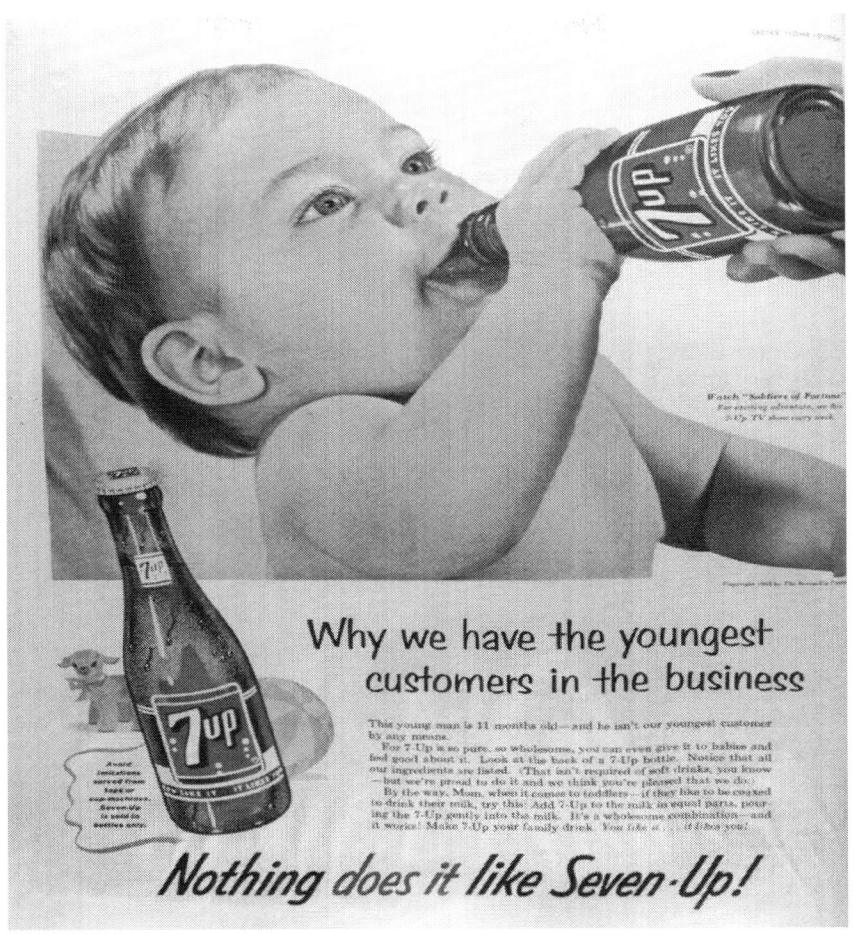

A would-be-funny-if-it-wasn't-so-sad example of deceptive 1955 advertising. Will we look back in 50 years with an equally ironic sophistication to Wendy's "You Know When It's Real" campaign, Nestle's "eco-shaped bottled water", and the other 98% of products world-wide tested in 2009 (by TerraChoice, who runs the Environmental Choice Program *for the Canadian government) whose labels were found to be misleadingly green-washed?*

Recently, the world's largest chain of natural food grocery stores, came under fire for misrepresenting the quality of their store-brand frozen organic vegetables. Turns out the "Organic California Blend", as well snap peas, spinach, and some others, were produced in China, and the store misleadingly and illegally put "USDA Organic" and "QAI" (Quality Assurance International) stamps on the foods, though neither organization had inspected the farms or food. They have, however, inspected hundreds of tons of food grown in China that were contaminated with chemicals and/or pathogens.

These stories shed light on the dark corners of the entire organic movement, which retailers like Whole Foods have ridden to massive financial success. Agriculture giants like Gerber's, Heinz, *Dole*, ConAgra and ADM, who have no problem poisoning workers, consumers, and the Earth with toxic chemical practices have jumped on the bandwagon with Earthy-friendly sounding organic subsidiaries. It takes little common sense to realize that massive conglomerates, who commonly purchase pesticides that have been outlawed in the US to use in their South American plants before shipping them back to American consumers (a bizarre loophole in the law), can't be trusted to make ethical decisions about my food when one simple lie can net them millions of dollars. Same goes for Target, recently sued for mislabeling natural products like rice milk and tofu as organic. Or that, though "organic farm" and "small family farm" are interchangeable in most consumer's minds,

> "If people let government decide what foods they eat, their bodies will soon be in as sorry a state as are the souls of those who live under tyranny." –Thomas Jefferson

almost all the organic food produced in America comes from California, where 5 or 6 huge operations dominate the market. 80% of US beef is produced by 4 companies[1]. The vast majority of the seeds planted by the world's farmers come from 4 conglomerations of companies. Food retailers are also on a consolidation track, and by some estimates, in the next ten years all of the retail food in the world will be controlled by 6 companies, only one of which will be American, Wal-Mart. Represent! This means that the selection and labeling of products on your grocery store shelves will be decided by a broker, potentially on another continent, based on what will return the largest profit.

If you sprout and grow your own food, you know it's organic. If you buy it, you only hope it is.

Home growing, sprouting, and fermenting is one of the best way to take responsibility for your own health and impact on the environment, and creates a haven from the conspiracy of corporate greed and consumer manipulation that plays like a Hollywood movie. The few seconds it takes to rinse our sprouts can re-establish our primordial bond to the land, the elements, and the moment-to-moment birth, maturation, and transformation of the pulsating forces of life around us. Even 100 glass and steel stories above the cement, life presses powerfully on. All this from an unused square-foot spot on a kitchen counter or closet shelf that would otherwise be collecting dust or worse, historical spoons from ebay.

---

[1] Nebraska and S Dakota passed constitutional amendments banning all farms not family-owned. Corporate agri-business didn't like that one bit, but state constitutions (and government in general) are in fact of, by, and for the people. Oops.

Collapse, the Future of Food

> "A living planet is a much more complex metaphor for deity than just a bigger father with a bigger fist. If an omniscient, all-powerful Dad ignores your prayers, it's taken personally. Hear only silence long enough, and you start wondering about his power. His fairness. His very existence. But if a world mother doesn't reply, Her excuse is simple. She never claimed conceited omnipotence. She has countless others clinging to her apron strings, including myriad species unable to speak for themselves. To Her elder offspring She says – 'Go raid the fridge. Go play outside. Go get a job. Or, better yet, lend me a hand. I have no time for idle whining.'" - David Brin, physicist and sci-fi writer

At a certain point, the rate of global extraction of crude petroleum products is reached, after which the rate of production enters a terminal decline. This is called "Peak Oil", and is another reason to become self-sustainable sooner than later. This is to say that there will come a day when our oil use will surpass the oil that's left in the ground, heading us towards the inevitable moment when there's no more left to power our cars and homes, our electric plants, to make our fertilizers and pesticides, or to run our farm equipment or the trucks that bring us the food.

Let's talk again about how commercial farms work. A field is fertilized, and all commercial fertilizers are made from ammonium nitrate, which is made from natural gas. This is sprayed onto the fields by an oil-powered machine. Another oil-powered machine ploughs, and another comes by and plants. The fields are irrigated with pumps powered by electricity, which comes from coal or, you guessed it: natural gas. But wait, there's more - oil-powered crop dusters spray oil-derived pesticides, once, twice, thrice. Then, when it's time to harvest, one oil-powered machine cuts, another loads, and another takes it to where it'll be processed by electric contraptions, and it's wrapped in plastic (made of oil) and trucked to a distribution center, then to the store. You can take it from there. There are 10 calories of hydrocarbon energy in every one calorie of food produced this way. Imagine that there's a finite amount of oil in the world and you'll soon realize that this would be a blatantly unsustainable system. Unfortunately, we'll soon be forced to see the end of this strategy.

Oil is made from the fossilized bodies of microorganisms, a process that takes millions of years. As of this writing, half of all the oil in the world has been used. The remaining half is of increasingly lower quality, and will require more and more energy to extract and refine. Oil is finite. Natural gas is finite, coal, uranium; all non-renewable energy sources are finite. There will be a peak for all of them. We're using, in a few decades, energy resources that took the planet millions of years to produce. Right now we are consuming 5 barrels of oil for every 1 barrel discovered.

> "Our agriculture system is almost wholly dependent on cheap fuel. Tremendous amounts of diesel fuel that are used in planting, and harvesting, and then, moving the stuff all these vast distances." - James Howard Kunstler *The Long Emergency*

For as long as I can remember, just about everyone I knew consumed like there was no tomorrow. My family threw away more food than many families in developing countries had. Now, when some of us in the West are just beginning to wake up to the realities of our wasteful lifestyle choices, those that have looked on hungrily for decades are starting to be able to enjoy the ease and luxury of modern life. In 1993, China had three quarters of a million cars on the road. At the start of 2004 they had 6 million, and in now (2010) they have 24 million. They idea behind a "developing" country is that one day they'll be able to consume like a first world country; they'll be able to live like the people in the movies. But this is clearly impossible. Even Americans in the near future won't be able to consume like Americans today.

Most of us have our heads in the sand about this to one degree or another; we know there's a problem looming but we're hoping that if we bring our own bags to the supermarket it'll go away. But the average person in a developed country can't really be blamed; with the demands of modern life, most people are happy with just a few minutes a day to relax and enjoy the life they're working so hard for. We've never had a peak in resources before and we have blinders on about it. Like statistics about climate change or overpopulation on a piece of paper, it's not an idea we can easily digest. We need new role models.

Peak Oil Pioneers

From 1950 to 1990, Cuba lived comfortably under Soviet communist care. Then, with little warning in 1991, the Soviet Union collapsed and Cuba's access to oil dropped to less than 25%. Everything changed in a matter of weeks. Suddenly, malnourished children, anemic pregnant women, and underweight babies became commonplace. The impact on food production and availability was disastrous. The average Cuban lost 20 pounds. Massive blackouts made refrigeration difficult so the little food that was available would often spoil. Cubans had to wait 3 to 4 hours for a bus to take them to school or work, and when it came it was often full, so they'd have to wait another 3 to 4 for the next one. And when they finally got to work, there might be no power, or no materials for them to do their jobs.

Then in 1992, the 30-year-old American embargo of Cuba was tightened. Before, companies were prohibited from doing business with both communist Cuba and the freedom-defending USA. Now, any ship even docking in a Cuban port was denied access to the US for 6 months afterwards. Almost overnight 750 million dollars worth of food and medical supplies pulled up anchor and sailed away. Then in 1996, the stranglehold was intensified. Cuba abruptly found itself with almost no access to foreign resources. The American dollar was worth 150 pesos, and the average daily salary was 20 pesos. Cubans was making about 4 dollars a month, so money was no longer a commodity that could be used to acquire the basics of life. A recently comfortable society abruptly found themselves cut-off, destitute, and hungry.

> "So we had now been like an experiment, with controlled conditions... Nothing, or very little... could get in from the outside, so everything had to happen from the inside." - Roberto Perez, Cuban permaculturist and educator, from documentary film *The Power of Community*

Every aspect of Cuban life was affected, but none more potently than farming. Before the collapse, Cuba's agriculture was more industrialized than any other Latin American country. It used a massive amount of fossil fuel for fertilizer, pesticides, farm machinery, and transportation - 2 or 3 times more than any other Latin American country, and acre for acre it surpassed the US in fertilizer consumption. Their farms had high yields, but these were in huge single-crop operations like tobacco, sugarcane, and citrus, which were exported while the basics were imported. The system wasn't set up to feed the people.

So the people: doctors, engineers, and lawyers, started sowing seeds in open places, without knowing how, because they were starving and there was no end in sight. The older generation, those that remembered how to operate a plough, how to tell if soil was acidic or alkaline by rolling it around in their mouths, were suddenly a valuable resource. A movement to use every arable piece of local land for growing food began. Every park, front yard, school, and vacant lot in Havana became a garden or orchard because there was no gas to transport food. And because there were no fossil fuels to produce chemical pesticides and fertilizers, over the months and seasons the fledgling farmers learned to use natural, organic pesticides like bugs and companion plants. Organic fertilizers like manure and compost were all they had.

They found ways to replenish the depleted soil with cheap and available resources, and to do their farming without the use of machinery. They used worms to turn sandy, dead soil into lush and nutrient-rich fertile ground. They found that they could extend the growing season by putting a fiber mesh between the plants and the sun, which would also control pests and was easily replaceable during hurricane season. As time went on, Cuban urban farmers found infinite small solutions to improve their lives. They dealt with the myriad complex problems that come with a new kind of agronomy by trial and error, and thrived. Formerly larger farms were divided up and leased to citizens for free by the government and the 2.2 million residents of Havana fed themselves from these rooftop gardens, schoolyard nurseries, and small farms within a few kilometers from the city.

Today, urban gardens in small Cuban cities and towns are even more productive, providing 80-100% of the residents' food, and over 80% of Cuba's food production is organic. In the 1980's Cuba used 21,000 tons of chemical pesticides per year; now they use less than 1000. Good for the soil, good for the environment, good for the economy, and great for the people.

Now, apartment-dwellers with a well laid-out porch, rooftop, or patio garden improve their lives by both cutting back on their food spending and selling their produce or homemade products like wine. Cuba's 140,000 urban farmers aren't the poorest people in society, as they are in many countries, like America, where farmers are constantly forced to cut corners and take the chemical way out. They are among the highest-paid professionals in the country, and are even exporting their natural pesticides, fertilizers, and knowledge to other countries. This rewarding occupation attracts people from all walks of life who don't want to be dependent on others for their sustenance. They have the respect of their communities and dignity of working in what has become one of the noblest professions.

The country as a whole is enjoying a slew of fringe benefits as well. They developed bio-organic farming methods because at the time they had no other choice. But now, with less than 2% of the population of Latin America, Cuba has 11% of its scientists. At the start of the

> "It wasn't the *Exxon Valdez* captain's driving that caused the Alaskan oil spill. It was yours." - Greenpeace advertisement, 1990

"Special Period", the name for Cuba's quiet revolution starting with the collapse of the Soviet Union, Cuba had 3 universities. It now has about 50, with 7 in Havana alone. Cuba's urban farmers produce much more from the same amount of land as their corporate counterparts and many of them donate a portion of their crops to the elderly, day-care centers and schools, orphanages, and pregnant women. They do this for free with no government involvement, because they want their community to thrive. Small farmers form co-ops, if they wish, to buy in bulk and share machinery. In many cities in richer countries, we don't even *know* our neighbors.

Cuba has roughly the same life expectancy and infant mortality rate as the US, though the average citizen uses 1/8th the energy and resources of the average American. They were once forced to be frugal with their energy consumption, using the sun to pre-heat cooking water, for example, but now it's a way of life. Why do most American homes have their hot-water heaters in cold closets and basements, requiring more fossil fuels to heat them, instead of outside in the sun? Sugar mills, which produce gas when the fibers are heated, are used as power plants, which now provide the country with 30% of its energy during harvest seasons. Increased walking and biking improved Cubans' fitness and drastically reduced diabetes (51% less deaths attributed to diabetes since before the Soviet collapse), heart disease (35% less), and strokes (20% less, and 18% less deaths overall). Cuba trains more doctors than they need, more than double the number of physician-to-citizen ration as America, and sends the surplus to developing countries around the world. Urban planners from all over the world study Havana as a model of livability. 85% of Cubans own their own home. The countryside, which has been called the last romantic place on earth, looks like a science-fiction comic book come alive with solar cells home-spun shacks, country school and rural hospitals. Cuba has reclaimed its health, its communities, its ethos, and its future.

The fact that Cuba is still looking for oil off their shores may surprise some. But unlike the vampires in developed countries that will start wars and enslave weaker nations for the life-blood of their consumer culture, they don't use what they find. If Cuba does hit upon the Texas tea, they sell it to wealthier countries at a premium, because they how to get by without it. We can wait until our own energy crisis to enact sustainable practices, and certainly the GOP government and their "head in the sand" policy-making will wait until it's too late. Or we can make changes now while we have some breathing room?

The concept of peak oil brings up another, much bigger question: what will happen to us when the greasy lubricant of our society becomes too expensive to be a viable means of energy?

Easter Island's Last Lumberjack

Easter Island is a remote dot of earth about 1500 miles off the coast of Chile. It's so small you can walk around the whole thing in a day. It's also the hauntingly desolate remains of a once-thriving civilization that numbered over 10,000 people.

When Easter Island was settled by 20 or 30 Polynesians halfway through the first millennium, it was a

> "There is a sufficiency in the world for man's need but not for man's greed." – Mahatma Gandhi

lush forest. The sweet potatoes and other crops the settlers brought with them thrived in the rich soil, living was easy, and the Easter Islanders found themselves with lots of free time. In about 1000 years, they swelled to a burgeoning society, and one of the most technologically advanced in the asncient world. Crops were protected by complex rock formations, and by some accounts every rock on the island was moved at least 3 or 4 times. The island's famous 600 stone statues, many of which were in sophisticated astronomical alignment, weighed tens of tons and were transported by human force, often for several miles over forested, hilly terrain. Each monument was laboriously carved from different color rock from quarries all over the island so the leaders of the clans could ask for favors from the Gods, and for a while it seemed to be working. But when European explorers reached the island in 1722, they found an arid grassland with less than 2000 malnourished people, many of whom had become cannibals, living in squalid reed huts and constant warfare. The explorers couldn't fathom how such a primitive society could be responsible for the socially and technologically advanced monuments, and because the island was nowa barren prairie, the transportation of behemoth idols seemed impossible. When asked how the 20-foot-high stone gods had gotten there, the inhabitants, wholly disconnected from their history, replied simply, "They walked".

Actually, the statues were pushed along rolling roads made of the island's trees, chopped down in huge swathes to make way for the huge stone carvings and laid side-by-side through miles of forest. The trees, which provided shelter, canoes for fishing, and fuel, were so abundant at the time that they could be used without fear of running out. But as the population continued to swell, and more and more clans were formed with more leaders, all needed their own statues lest their dependants miss out on their slice of the divine benevolence pie and the ability to live as well as their neighbors. Competition for resources between clans grew fierce, and then someone, one day, cut down the last tree on the island. No more boats for fishing. No more fuel for heat, cooking, or transporting statues. The topsoil eroded at a breakneck pace and the gravely land couldn't hold in moisture or nutrients. Hundreds of great stone deities were abandoned, unfinished, in quarries around the islands. The gods were not happy. With no logs for buildings, people began living in caves and flimsy reed huts, fiercely protecting their meager assets. Cannibalism became a reasonable means of dealing with both enemies and hunger. Like the Romans, Byzantines, Vikings, and Mayans before them, the Easter Islanders didn't think total collapse happen to them, and lived recklessly until it did.

> "We never know the worth of water till the well is dry." - Thomas Fuller, *Gnomologia*, 1732

The pattern is clear. When civilizations over-consume, they cut off the legs of their own life-support systems and begin to fight each other over what little is left. Then they either starve or leave. Our current problems are global: climate change, overpopulation, peak oil, genetically manipulated genes out-crossing into the DNA of the world's food supply; so there's nowhere to go, just like boatless Easter Islanders on a remote island in the middle of the Pacific. We can't abandon our planet and set off for a new Eden. We're here, and we have only two choices: cut down the last tree, or take an objective look at the dilemmas facing our species as a whole, and find another way to live.

A very early action of the Bush administration upon assuming office in 2001 was to lobby for the replacement of the chairman of the official United Nations Intergovernmental Panel on Climate Change (IPCC). This was done at the request of Exxon, who felt the sitting chairman, Dr. Watson, was too "aggressive" in pursuing action on the issue of global warming. As a result of actions taken by the administration, Dr. Watson was replaced ("at the request of the US") by the industry-friendly Dr. Rajendra Pachauri, hand-picked by the administration, and referred to by former vice-president Al Gore as the "let's drag our feet" candidate. Four years later, Dr. Pachauri issued the strongest warning yet in regard to global climate change, and a most urgent call for immediate action. His report stated that there is not a moment to lose, and added that we are risking the ability of the human race to survive. He called for "very deep" cuts in current pollution levels, stating that the point of no return was rapidly approaching.

> "The American way of life is non-negotiable" - Dick Cheney

Sometimes big change comes through a big effort. But more often, revolution is the result of very small actions repeated over time. For a while, maybe for several generations, the results of our efforts are almost unnoticeable, but then there comes a "tipping point" where the slow incremental change has completely reshaped society. It's like driving. Turn the wheel dramatically and you find yourself on the beginning of a different road, or in a ditch. But turn the wheel just 5 degrees, and for a while it seems like nothing's different. Then, after enough miles, the car is in a completely different place, a totally different course. This is the way to lasting change, to guaranteed metamorphosis. When someone wants a major turn-around in their health, for example, I always recommend making one small change a day. In a year, they'll have made 365 little improvements, which adds up to a big difference. And they'll have made new habits and the stamina to maintain them, encouraged by the changes they notice in their life, how they feel, etc. I encourage treating anything important as a marathon, not a sprint, and diging in for the long haul.

It's true that massive change is overdue: in the way we treat each other, our world, and ourselves. But I don't have the dynamite nor a flair for drama. Instead, I just make one improvement at a time, stabilize it, and then see where I'm at. I've gotten excited and gung-ho about a lot of things in my life, but I've noticed that permanent and powerful transformation has come about from a sustained 5% turn of the wheel. If you're different, that's awesome, together I hope we can make something really magical happen.

> "Greater than the tread of mighty armies is *an idea whose time has come*." - Victor Hugo

Everyone but the Kitchen Sink: Modernization, McDonald's, and Hyper-Maturation

I'd like to make it clear that this book is for absolutely everyone. The ways of making and preparing food in here aren't just for already-organic urban yoga hipster families; they're for the low-income families that can't afford fresh vegetables, communities and aid-workers in developing countries, and the one-third of American kids that eat fast food every day.

Evolution is slow; it certainly can't keep up with the modernization of our diets. Our Paleolithic hunter-gatherer ancestors lived on hundreds of different wild plant sources, some meat (in the few climates where killing a creature that was running or fighting for its life was less effort than foraging for edible plants), and thereby guaranteed themselves a vast array of potent, living nutrients. Just to put it in perspective, of the food crops grown in 1900, 97% were extinct in 2000, just a hundred years later. And we're talking about the vast changes in lifestyle over the course of half a million years, while our basic biology has stayed the same. In the prehistoric world, starch, fat, and salt were rare commodities that our brains were programmed to seek out with the fervor of junkies. Now, they are available on every street corner in the developed world, and the fast food "restaurants" that offer them claim different characteristics and even different cultures, starch, fat, and salt are found in almost every case in the precise proportions that mirror the cravings imprinted in our very genes, with lab-concocted cocktails of smells pumped into the air to lure our Paleolithic minds in the door.

Ten thousand years ago (a time frame too short to cause many genetic changes, though one exception is the continued production of lactase, the milk enzyme, in about 25% of post-nursing humans), our ancestors went from a wild food diet totally free of grains to an agricultural lifestyle, in a move that author and UCLA Professor of Physiology Dr. Jared Diamond calls "The Worst Mistake in the History of the Human Race" in his essay of the same name. Our forefathers began growing not the crops that would protect the delicate balance of their health and longevity, but the ones that were the easiest to cultivate, harvest, and store: wheat, rice, and corn began providing the most calories to humanity. The average lifespan promptly dropped seven years[2].

---

[2] Pia Bennike, *Paleopathology of Danish Skeletons* [Copenhagen: Almquist and Wiskell, 1985]; and N-G Gejvall, *Westerhu: Medeviel Populations and Church in the Light of Skeletal Remains* [Lund: Hakan Ohlssons Boktryckeri, 1960]

It's no surprise that we're not cut out for the amount of starch, salt and particularly fat in our diet, as it's quickly killing us; heart disease, diabetes, and cancer are all linked to a diet too high in these foods. McDonalds lost two CEOs in a single year to diet-related diseases (2004): heart attack and colon cancer[3]. The majority of Americans are on at least one prescription drug to treat type-2 diabetes, cholesterol, and high blood pressure, all of which are directly related to starch, fat, or salt.

Less lethal but just as alarming are the effects of diets high in trans- and saturated fats on children. The number of overweight children has tripled in the last three decades. Kid's menus at sit-down restaurants are usually much worse than the adults'. Our schools are "7-11's with books" (Yale diet expert Kelly Brownell). Shortened and less happy lives will be the obvious result, but there are more nefarious effects as well. Throughout most of our species' history, female sexual maturity was reached at 17 ½ to 18 years old. In 1900, the age had dropped to 15 ½ in developed countries, and now the average age that girls reach puberty is 11, while many girls mature sexually at 9 or 10. Many researchers originally believed this accelerating change was due to ingesting the hormones given to milk cows and meat animals to speed *their* maturation and growth, but recent studies show that the single greatest cause is the estrogenic effect of additional fat cells in the girls' bodies. Boys show a much less dramatic change, putting them far out of sync with the girls, with the exception of the most overweight boys whose puberty is actually slowed down by the increased estrogen

---

[3] I'd like to add, however, that the second CEO, Australian Charile Bell, perhaps prompted by the release of the documentary film Super Size Me criticizing the health of McDonald's food, led efforts to add healthier choices to the McDonald's menu and offered parents the option to substitute juice and apple slices for fries and soft drinks for their children. The "Supersize" option was also eliminated.

in their body fat. One result of living out of harmony with our biology.

Cultural awareness of the alarming health problems has been steadily growing over the past decade. Ten years ago the public acknowledged that we were in the throes of a losing battle with obesity and heart disease. Two-thirds of Americans were overweight. Obesity-related illnesses killed a third of a million people every year, crippling millions, and costing our health care system almost a hundred billion dollars annually. Overwhelmingly, people singled out their excess weight as the thing they most disliked about their bodies.

In the past ten years, Americans have made a number of choices about their diet and health. The average America has eaten 50% *more* fast food meals and 5 more pounds of sugar per year. Hospital bills related to obesity have risen to $117 billion, and it's estimated that 8 out of 10 Americans are or will become overweight.

In 2004, the World Health Organization proposed dietary guidelines to reduce fat and sugar consumption. The US delegation, which represents the fattest nation in the world, protested these changes, on behalf of the food industry, as "scientifically unproven". While the WHO guidelines call on governments to reduce the unhealthy food advertising aimed at children and use fiscal incentives to limit the availability of junk food and amount of trans fats in the diet, the US Department of Health and Human Services responded that it would be best to use tactics like "better data and surveillance, and the promotion of sustainable strategies that focus on energy balance," hollow and meaningless expressions with just enough buzzwords to dupe the most foolish into thinking that something was being done.

Former senator Peter Fitzgerald noted that putting the USDA, whose first job it is to sell agricultural products, in charge of our dietary guidelines was like "putting a fox in charge of the hen house". The USDA subsidizes farmers to grow high-calorie, low nutrition crops for $19 billion annually, making white flour, corn syrup, hydrogenated margarine, and white rice cost sometimes less than nothing to produce. It becomes these foods that are the most heavily-advertised and make up the bulk of ingredients of fast food, junk food, and school lunches. And while the current administration is offering small subsidies to farms that convert to organic methods, an initiative spearheaded by Mrs. Obama (who is taking much of the ill-placed heat from farmers losing their hard-won handouts) , still not a penny goes towards large-scale vegetable farming. I've gone into such detail in these last few paragraphs to illuminate the fact that the very government agencies we've put in place to protect our health and well-being can't be counted on to do that very thing. It is, once again, up to us to take responsibility for our own health.

But it's difficult to choose fresh food when $5 feeds a busy family at McDonald's. Fast and junk food are designed to maximize the cheapest ingredients, and grocery stores can rarely compete. Add to that the time it takes to shop for and prepare dinner and it becomes a daunting task for haggard parents. But an even less expensive meal, both in money and in medical bills, can be had with a deep breath, a few minutes' forethought, and the application of the methods in this book, in even less time than it takes to round up the kids and drive to the transfat pusher on the corner with a winning goatee and bowtie or cute red pigtails. While the dangers of not making a change in our families' diets could be their own encyclopedia, the benefits of doing so are simple: turning our children into vivacious young people with strong immune systems, increased focus and learning - the kids they were meant to be. It's my fervent desire that the mostly unoriginal ideas presented in these books will spread not only to the families that can most easily implement them, but to the ones that need them most.

Changing Food Habits - Using the Brain for a Change

I doubt that the previous section is enough to shock people into changing their diets. We all know what to do to be healthier: eat more vegetables and less crap, exercise. It's usually not the why nor the what that holds us up, but the how. Willpower or self-talk alone isn't enough to make lasting changes for most people, and just like the force that drives us to continue eating the ice cream our conscious minds know we've had enough of, the reason is our wiring.

The human brain is "an organ so complex we may never fully understand it", says Colin Blakemore, British neurobiologist. There are 100 billion nerve cells in the brain, with ten thousand times as many connections between them. On average, our brains make one million data transfers every second, for the entirety of our lifetimes. Recent studies have found brain cells previously thought to exist only inside our skulls are actually dispersed throughout our entire bodies, amplifying the previous number by orders of magnitude.

In addition to being the miraculous instrument of human achievement, according to David Linden, a professor of neuroscience at Johns Hopkins University the brain is a "cobbled-together mess... quirky, inefficient and bizarre ... a weird agglomeration of ad hoc solutions that have accumulated throughout millions of years of evolutionary history," he states in his book, "The Accidental Mind," from Harvard University Press. Interestingly, when new kingdoms of species evolved: reptiles to mammals, lower mammals to humans, the brain didn't actually evolve. The entire reptilian brain stayed almost as is, and a new brain was added on top. That means that we're all carrying around the brains of a flatworm, a snake and a primate right next to our advanced thinking capabilities.

The reptilian area of the brain governs habits and emotions and will always choose the easy route if left to its own, literally subconscious, devices. Specifically, the basal ganglia (BG) is a loosely grouped collection of nerve cells located deep within the reptilian part of each cerebral hemisphere. It's responsible for rage, fear, love, lust, contentment, and automatic behaviors like slamming on the brakes, smashing a vase against a wall in startling anger, or opening the fridge to grab the cheesecake before you even know you're doing it. The pre-frontal cortex (PFC) is the newest addition to the human brain, situated right behind the forehead and is in charge of the things that make us human: personality and executive functions: goal-setting, understanding consequences, and differentiating between conflicting thoughts to choose (hopefully) the most enlightened course of action. Basically, it's considered to be the conscious conductor in the orchestration of thoughts and actions in accordance with internal goals. The BG pushes for habitual behavior, while the PFC considers whether or not that deed is going to bring us what we want in the long run. An over-simplified example of this is the drug-addicted brain, which tells the owner in increasingly creative ways that more drugs are needed. We know as observers that the best course of action is to re-shape the desires of the BG by stopping the drug use and consequently changing the messages being sent to the PFC, but just like an addict's brain invents evidence to show that more drug use is the best course of action, within the individual an entirely different story is told.

An iguana or python doesn't respond to coaxing, cajoling, or bargaining; it changes its habits based on repetition, pure and simple. The ritualistic nature of this organ leaves no room for complex emotions (my apologies to the shirtless-under-their-leather-vests guys at the beach with their scaly loved ones.) The time it takes to change a habit depends on how ingrained it is. It's a simple formula. When a wagon wheel goes over the same road, in the same way, an ever-deepening rut results. If the wheel happens to find new ground, all it takes is a little push in the same old direction and the wheel teeters then returns to the rut. But push in a new direction everyday and the wheel will in no time make a new groove, soon becoming deeper than the first and the wheel will easily stay into it, propelling the cart effortlessly in a new direction. Absolutely any habit can change from a rut to a groove, given enough pushes. Research states that simple habits take 21 days to break, and while we're dealing with more complicated lifestyle changes, 3 weeks of daily action and at least the beginnings of changes are guaranteed. If it's a worthwhile goal, these incremental encouragements may, like signposts on the proverbial road, be all that's needed to propel you towards lasting change. It all starts with one action, today.

The pleasure mechanism in the human brain is *extremely* flexible. It will attach to whatever is introduced, whether unconsciously, like heroin or Big Macs, or consciously like whole living foods. We can quite literally re-engineer our evolution, rewire our brains. The brain of someone who has made a habit of a simple sprout salad with homemade vinaigrette will release just as much dopamine, the "pleasure chemical", as a steak and potatoes guy will get from his 20-oz ribeye. The satisfaction of improving our health and the self-esteem that results is enough to pull back the veil of denial that results in actions that destroy ourselves, other creatures, and the planet, and we will soon have a network of habits and beliefs that will make it easy for us to make better choices.

I know from personal experience. As I slowly started eating more and more whole, living, simple foods, I was surprised to find myself craving whole, living, simple foods. If you've never jones-ed after raw baby spinach, it is a pretty wonderful feeling. Processed food started looking like wax fruit, (eg - not food), and non-organic food had an unmistakably flat and empty taste. When I travel, I try to sprout as much food as possible and I obviously lean towards authentic and clean cuisines, especially in places like Germany where GMOs are outlawed and almost all the food is grown with traditional organic methods. It's not always possible or polite to eat this way, however and after a month or two of bratwurst, potato salad, and strudel and the impulses coming from my BG have become quite distorted. It takes just a few meals to start affecting unconstructive change, and about 3-4 times as long to re-position positive habits in the BG. I don't know why negative transformation seems to have more pull than the other direction, but when I get back home I'm bolstered by the fact that the challenging choices I face will soon become effortless, and because of the nature of the basal ganglia-pre-frontal cortex connection, dramatic changes in behavior can make it even easier. Humans have the largest PFC of any animal. Let's put it to use for a better life now and a brighter future for the planet.

Transitioning to a Living Diet

When we're used to cooked food, we usually look for one thing out of our meals, besides the immediate taste sensations: a "feeling of fullness". Living foods nourish our bodies in a completely different, and much more thorough way. This become clear to me during a recent dinner I prepared for some friends and family where one person refused to eat the meal, worrying that they were sure they "wouldn't get filled up from it". That relation grabbed a sandwich from a nearby convenience store and scarfed the fistful of spongy white bread and deli meats while the rest of us enjoyed a living meal. Afterwards, I noticed the general ebullience of the family and the heavy, lethargic quality of that individual. Granted, their food choice may have been healthier if they hadn't had to scrounge for dinner after being ambushed by an alfalfa-weilding hippie, but it's an interesting dichotomy. The "fill your belly", "stick to your ribs" mentality is quite the opposite of being fed on a cellular level, really nourished down to the nerve, where the energy that used to go into digestion and assimilation are already in the food and don't need to be stolen from the body's other processes. It's a different kind of satiction with living food when you're used to heavy meats and caramelized starches, but in time you will adjust, if you choose to go that route.

Table 2: Seed/Nut Digestibility Chart

How	What	Why
Toasted	Starches (usually the main component) are caramelized and impossible to utilize. Most vitamins and minerals diminished or gone. Enzymes gone. Some oils are toxic.	Enzymes are destroyed over 108 degrees; most nutrients are destroyed at high temperatures. Heating some oils past 170 degrees creates free radicals and other toxins.1
Raw, right outta the bag	The most difficult to digest and assimilate; heating does destroy (denature the molecular bonds and render inert) some EI's.	Nutrients are in a dormant state and bound with EI's; these rob the body of its own enzymes and more effort than necessary is put into digestion, while less energy than possible is gotten out in nutrition. The living enzymes of the seed are dormant and unusable.
Soaked in water	Easier to handle, but not at peak nutrition.	Soaking starts the germination process, breaking down the EI's so they can be rinsed away, but enzymes aren't fully

		activated, nor are nutrients levels substantially increased, but you're on the right track...
Fermented (in probiotic water, miso, or seed cheese, for example)	Partial probiotic pre-digestion makes protein, healthy fats, vitamins, minerals, and starches present in dormant seed more available.	Beneficial microorganisms go to work on the starches and long-chain proteins, turning them into more easily-digestible simple sugars and amino acids, and thereby taking some of the strain off of the human. Blending with probiotic water releases EI's which are removed by bacteria.
Sprouted	Nutrient levels are at their peak, enzymes fully active. Provides the body with the building blocks of health and an abundance of energy with which to use them.	

| Sprouted and Fermented | Bacteria make immunity-supporting compounds you can't get anywhere else. Peak nutrition and complex components broken down into easily-assimilable forms. The benefits of the seed's inherent nutrition and life force, the short-term benevolent action of friendly bacteria on the seed and the long-term advantages to the digestive system as porbiotics settle in and prepare to convert everything that comes their way into a greater you. | Plus it tastes freaking awesome. |

The "How?"

Growing

Sprouts and Greens

Sprouts are a seed that's formed a tail, and we eat the entire thing. Greens are a sprout that's been taken a further step; its roots have burrowed into something that keeps it upright, and contains moisture and nutrients. Soil is one such thing and once the sprouts' roots have become one with the dirt, we eat just what's above. All leafy green sprouts can be grown in this manner: alfalfa, clover, watercress, broccoli, etc., and will become micro-lettuce, micro-greens, or nano-greens if they're really small. All of these are smaller than baby lettuces or greens, usually chopped at a couple of inches after 1-3 weeks. Grains such as wheat, rye, barley, and oats can be grown into grasses, which aren't great eaten straight but make ridiculously nutritious and cleansing juice. This section covers the next step of planting your sprout seeds in a shallow growing medium to take them to their next level, and the couple of things you'll need to have and know to do it.

Grass and Micro-Greens

Growing grasses and micro lettuces is somewhere in between sprouting and gardening. After seeds are sprouted in the normal way, they're transferred onto a tray filled with growing medium, which is either soil or man-made (though I'll show you how to skip one or both of those steps in some cases). Then they're rinsed and drained twice a day, aka "watered", just like sprouts, for a week or more. Lighting must be taken into consideration, because these more mature plants need chlorophyll to grow up strong, and their oxygenating greenness is a major health benefit of your developing crops. The little bit of effort that goes into planning the space, getting the materials and taking an extra step or two in growing will yield you diminutive fields of delicious salad greens and an unlimited supply of juice

which is "literally condensed sunlight energy. It is one of the most potent healing agents on the planet" (author Steve Meyerowitz,
Wheatgrass: Nature's Finest Medicine), for pennies.

Why Grow Grass?

In the early 1900's, Edmond Bordeaux Szekely, a linguist and philosopher who held several Ph.Ds and professorships was studying ancient texts at the Vatican. His laborious research uncovered four Aramaic and Hebrew volumes that would become the "Essene Gospels of Peace", manuscripts written by a sect of religious mystics that lived between 200 BC and 100 AD near the Dead Sea between present-day Jordan and Israel, and who were also responsible for the famous "Dead Sea Scrolls". A good chunk of these writings deal with the Essene's health practices, which were supposedly later taught to the abstinent ascetics by Jesus. In the books, the distribution of which became Szekely's life purpose, Jesus prescribes vegetarianism, eating living foods, and the benefits of grasses.

Though information about the use of grasses for human and animal health was available, it remained a fringe and esoteric knowledge until the 1940's, when future health pioneer Ann Wigmore cured her cancer with the wild grasses and weeds that grew in vacant lots near her home in Boston. After studying thousands of types of grasses, she and a physician colleague decided that a) all grasses are good for human and animal consumption, and b) wheatgrass was the best. Then in the mid-seventies, the Japanese owner of a pharmaceutical company, Dr. Yoshihide Hagiwara, became very sick from working with the drugs his company produced, many of which were his formulations. After several years of trying and failing to improve his health through medicine, he began looking into traditional Chinese medicine. There, he discovered the philosophy behind the writings of Shin Huang-ti, the father of Chinese medicine, who said: "It is the diet which maintains true health and becomes the best drug". Similarly, Hippocrates, the father of Western medicine advised, "Let your food be your medicine." After exhaustively studying over 150 plants during the course of 13 years, Dr. Hagiwara decided that barley grass was nature's most healing food and began to cure himself immediately.

"Green[s] should not be recognized by discussing the amount of [their] vitamins and minerals. The era of focusing on a single vitamin or mineral is gone...much more attention is being focused on biological phenomenon." - Dr. Yoshihide Hagiwara

"In a recent John Hopkins study, 95 percent of 200 arthritis patients found almost complete relief after taking two ounces of wheatgrass juice a day for three weeks. I can attest to this fact when witnessing a crippled lady unable to climb stairs do so in three weeks on wheatgrass juice and living food. In my own healing, my body has cleansed from toxins, I became emotionally sound, drug-free, had more energy, felt more self worth, lost weight and returned home to live a more fulfilling life." - Loretta Harmony Kohn, former employee at Ann Wigmore's Hippocrates Institute

The Benefits of Wheatgrass Grass Juice

Wheatgrass juice is one of the most mineral-rich foods on the planet, and one ounce of juice contains about as many nutrients as 2.5 pounds of green vegetables. It's a complete food and excellent source of vitamins, including B12, which is very hard to find in a vegan diet. It contains 17 amino acids and about 80 known enzymes.

Wheatgrass juice is also the highest food source of a nutrient called chlorophyll, which is the green pigment in plants that let them turn sunshine into energy.

The chlorophyll molecule is remarkably similar to hemoglobin in human blood, the substance that carries oxygen in our body. The only difference is that hemoglobin has an iron element in the center of the structure, which is red, and chlorophyll has a magnesium element, which is green.

Dr. Yoshihide Hagiwara, president of the Hagiwara Institute of Health in Japan, is a leading advocate for the use of grass as food and medicine. He reasons that since chlorophyll is soluble in fat particles, and fat particles are absorbed directly into the blood via the lymphatic system, that chlorophyll can also be absorbed in this way. In other words, when the "blood" of plants is absorbed in humans it is transformed into human blood, which transports nutrients to every cell of the body. Wheatgrass juice is like a liquid oxygen transfusion. Oxygen is vital to many body processes: it stimulates digestion (the oxidation of food), promotes clearer thinking (the brain utilizes 25% of the body's oxygen supply), and protects the blood against anaerobic bacteria. Cancer cells cannot exist in the presence of oxygen.

Wheatgrass is also the courier of many other benefits:

- It restores alkalinity to the blood. It has been used successfully to treat peptic ulcers, ulcerative colitis, constipation, diarrhea, and other complaints of the gastrointestinal tract. (see section on Alkalinity in "Kitchen Sink Farming Volume 1: Sprouting", pg 112)
- It increases red blood-cell count and lowers blood pressure. It cleanses the blood, organs and gastrointestinal tract of debris. Wheatgrass also stimulates metabolism and the body's enzyme production. It also aids in reducing blood pressure by dilating the blood pathways throughout the body, removing plaque build-up in the blood vessels and the sources of plaque.
- It stimulates the thyroid gland, correcting obesity, indigestion, and a host of other complaints.
- It is a powerful detoxifier, and liver and blood protector. The enzymes and amino acids found in wheatgrass can protect us from carcinogens like no other food or medicine. It strengthens our cells, detoxifies the liver and bloodstream, and chemically neutralizes environmental pollutants. Wheatgrass rejuvenates aging cells by cleansing the blood and helps slow the aging process. It will help tighten loose and sagging skin.
- It fights tumors and neutralizes toxins. Recent studies show that wheatgrass juice has a powerful ability to fight tumors without the usual toxicity of drugs that also inhibit cell-destroying agents. It neutralizes toxic substances like cadmium, nicotine, strontium, mercury, and polyvinyl chloride [PVC].
- It contains beneficial enzymes. Whether healing a cut or dissolving fat while you exercise, enzymes do the actual work. The life and abilities of the enzymes found naturally in our bodies can be extended if we help them from the outside by adding exogenous enzymes, like the ones found in wheatgrass juice. We can only get the benefits of

the many enzymes found in grass by eating it uncooked. Cooking destroys 100 percent of the enzymes in food.
- Applied to the skin, wheatgrass juice can help eliminate itching almost immediately. It will soothe sunburned skin and act as a disinfectant. Rubbed into the scalp before a shampoo, it will help mend damaged hair and alleviate itchy, scaly, scalp conditions. Is soothing and healing for cuts, burns, scrapes, rashes, poison ivy, athlete's foot, insect bites, boils, sores, open ulcers, tumors, and so on. Use the juice (or wet pulp) as a poultice and replace every two to four hours.
- It works as a sleep aid. Put a tray of living wheatgrass near the head of your bed as you sleep - it will enhance the oxygen in the air and generate healthful negative ions to help you sleep more soundly.
- It sweetens the breath and firms up and tightens gums. Just gargle and swish the juice before you swallow it.
- Because of it's powerful oxygenating properties, it can turn gray hair back to its natural color and greatly increase energy levels when consumed daily. It can also decrease or remove body odor, which is bacteria putrefying on partially digrsted wastes excreted through the skin and build up in places without much air flow, like armpits. In much the same way is can combat halitosis, or bad breath.
- One enzyme found in wheatgrass, SOD, lessens the effects of radiation and acts as an anti-inflammatory compound that may prevent cellular damage following heart attacks or exposure to irritants.
- Studies have shown wheatgrass to restore fertility in women and increase lactation.
- This is one of the very few juices that can actually remove heavy metals from the system. Regular

consumption will greatly help to prevent Alzheimer's disease and any other mental problems.
- It can double the red blood cell count just by soaking in it. Renowned nutritionist Dr. Bernard Jensen found that no other blood builders are superior to green juices and wheatgrass. In his book *Health Magic Through Chlorophyll from Living Plant Life* he mentions several cases where he was able to double the red blood cell count in a matter of days merely by having patients soak in a chlorophyll-water bath. Blood building results occur even more rapidly when patients drink green juices and wheatgrass regularly. Wheatgrass has been shown to build levels of iron in the body and thereby relieve anemia. It also helps balance blood sugar.
- The high anti-oxidant content helps neutralize free radicals and oxidation that find their way in the body. It helps reduce the harm caused by air pollutants like carbon monoxide or cigarette smoke.
- Health experts believe wheatgrass is effective in treating arthritis. Chlorophyll is thought to benefit arthritis and wheatgrass contains tons of it. Chlorophyll fights inflammation, which is associated with joint pain.
- When experiencing fatigue, the body is deprived of oxygen and has a weakened immune system. Chlorophyll helps to increase oxygen supply in the body's cells and tissues, contributing to cell regeneration, healing the body and reducing fatigue symptoms.
- The fine chlorophyll and beta-carotene obtained from wheatgrass juice is beneficial in fighting and preventing cancer. A variety of flavonoid compounds found in this grass are powerful anti-oxidants and anti-cancer agents. Studies have indicated at least a 40% risk reduction in cancer development.

- The anti-bacteria effect of wheatgrass creates an unfavorable environment for yeast and harmful bacteria (those that live without the precense of oxygen). Regular consumption of this juice will help to prevent further yeast (candida) and bacterial growth.

Nutritional Benefits

The most outstanding feature of wheatgrass juice is its very high content of chlorophyll, about 70%. This alone makes it a superfood that has a highly energizing and alkalizing effect.

But wheatgrass has many vitamins and minerals, and is an excellent source of vitamin C, E, K and B complex (including B12). In the minerals department, it is rich in calcium, cobalt, germanium, iron, magnesium, phosphorus, potassium, protein, sodium, sulphur, and zinc.

This miracle grass also has a long list of amino acids – about 17 types of them and about 80 known enzymes.

Why Cleansing is Important

Early 20th century French biologist Dr. Alexis Carrel was fascinated by the aging process, and hypothesized that cells could live much longer in a clean environment. In an experiment began in 1912, Carrel took cells from an embryonic chicken heart and suspended them in a saline solution of the proper pH, temperature, and nutrient balance. He changed this fluid daily, and the cells, which would normally die after a few months, lived for 28 years. The experiment was stopped because the results were conclusive: "The cell is immortal. It is merely the fluid in which it floats which degenerates. Renew this fluid at intervals, give the cells what they require for nutrition and, as far as we know, the pulsation of life may go on forever." – Dr. Alexis Carrel, winner of the Nobel Prize in Medicine for this experiment.

The cleansing and waste removal systems of our body: the digestive system, bloodstream, liver, lymph, lungs, skin, and others, become clogged with toxins over time, impairing the normal functioning of all body processes. Short-term cleanses that target each of these systems are an important aspect of over-all health and well-being. But the most powerful and effective cleanse is the one that happens every day, in every cell, in every system of our bodies; the purification and rebuilding that our bodies do automatically when given the proper nutrients. I came across the Alexis Carrel experiment when I was very young, and I've been doing cleanses for most of my life. In addition to a diet and lifestyle fairly well free of toxins, I've done all the organ- and system-specific cleanses I could find. Having my body is the only thing that's certain throughout my life, and its condition is the number one factor that effects my happiness. So I try to take better care of it than redneck does his truck. We don't assume that our cars will fix themselves if we ignore a clunking sound or flat tire, but our bodies are such powerful machines of cleansing and regeneration that's just how we treat them. The most powerful cleanse I've ever done, or rather experienced, is the one that happened when I started eating only living foods. There are subtle shifts and pendulous swings one notices when doing a cleanse: no appetite giving way to ravenous hunger, almost overwhelming amounts of energy cycling with wanting to sleep for 12 hours a night, laser-like focus alternating with an impenetrable mental fog. These symptoms in the presence of top-quality nutrition and mechanisms of detoxification are a sign that the body's innate wisdom sees an opportunity to get rid of accumulated toxins, which were formerly rushed out of the bloodstream and into the safety of fat deposits to be dealt with only if a healthy opportunity presented itself. When I started on nutrient-rich living food that I grew myself, these cycles continued for about 6 months, in a slowly spiraling upward trend towards a newfound vitality that I had previously only wistfully imagined. More energy and better sleeping, fresher breath and a more positive outlook, brighter eyes and skin; the benefits that are commonly associated with cleansing were just the beginning. And it was health problems that made me make the change, not already glowing health that I was fine-tuning. It's as if I was building an entirely new body, optimal vehicle for my life force given my age and genetics.

I'll wrap up the section on cleansing with one more quote, credited to Eubie Blake, jazz and ragtime pianist who lived from 1883 to 1983:

"If I'd known I was going to live this long, I would have taken better care of myself."

Take care of yourself.

FURTHERMORE

As in the Dr. Hagiwara quote above, trying to understand a single nutrient, even one as potent as chloryphyll, is limiting in scope. The ICP (inductively coupled plasma) spectrometer, an imaging device about the size of a pickup truck, shows us that food nutrients are more varied and numerous that we ever imagined. A grape, for example, contains over 5 million compounds. Modern science has barely scratched the surface of comprehending or even naming these nutrients, let alone understanding the seemingly infinite interactions between them. And while single nutrients are important and we have to go with the info that we have when treating disease or discomfort, it seems silly to rely on such a fractured approach to nourishment. The best vitamins are whole, living foods, pulled directly from the dirt, or vine, or branch, that have been proven for centuries or millennia to repair and maintain vibrant human health.

How to Grow and Enjoy Grasses

To grow grain seeds into cleansing and nutritious grasses, they must be soaked, sprouted, then taken one step further. After they've grown a small tail, they are transferred onto a tray of growing media, where their little roots have an opportunity to take hold and support the development of bright green blades, they will shoot upwards like, well, grass. For this, you'll need a couple of extra tools: dirt or a dirt substitute, and something to hold it in. We'll also be discussing light, plant food, and because we're growing it for 2 weeks or more, pests in the form of molds, fungi, and bugs.

Dirt, New and Used

"Growing media" is the names of the various things seeds can be planted in, and serve three purposes: holding the plants up, retaining moisture, and most importantly, providing nutrients to the growing plants. Supporting most grass and micro-greens is easy; in fact, in just a couple of days many plants will quickly create their own thick mat of interwoven roots. With 2 or 3 daily waterings, the plants can stay moist enough, but when I tried many times to grow grass this way to try and save my apartment-bound readers the extra effort of dealing with dirt, the grass was always weakly and eventually taken over by mold and fungus. When planted on dirt, however, the same sprouts yielded strong, bright green blades of healthy and darkly emerald juice. So though it's possible to grow a bed of grass or micro-lettuce without any more support than its roots and neighbors provide, I recommend using growing media of some kind, the practical varieties of which are described.

Dirt

As the weeds growing up through cracks in a city sidewalk will maintain, any soil will work for growing grasses and micro-lettuce. Organic is always better, and some retail soils contain beneficial microbes which will create an environment of more available nutrients for your plants. Most store-bought soils don't have these microbial helpers or advertise the microorganisms they do contain, so a sterile soil will yield a more reliable growing material. Obviously, dirt is also available for free in most of the world. Composted cow manure or earthworm castings make a dark, loamy soil full of nutrients for your grass to thrive on, and is often given away by gardeners and farmers. It's also the stuff underneath the grass in city parks. I don't know your local laws (heck, I don't even know mine) but I recommend you check them before you head to the park with a shovel. For growing grasses, dirt can be used only once, as the afore-mentioned root matting will turn it into a solid carpet. For most micro-greens, which have a less tenacious root structure than grass, soil can be turned it over, fertilized, and used again for another crop. Then compost the whole thing or take it back to the park or woods you got it from, and with the addition of your organic fertilizer and plant matter, the returning soil will be better than you found it. Choose soil from out-of-the-way places, avoiding places that are walked or peed on if possible. The base of a tree is bound to have nutrient-rich, biologically active soil, as the tree roots protect it from both mineral erosion and pathogens.

Dealing with dirt in an apartment

Soil is great because it is (or can be) free and renewable, not in the grand scheme of things but in your own yard or city park, but it's also the only growing medium that has its own built-in nutrients and for this reason it's my #1 choice. Dirt is a living, breathing thing, and supports more life within than on top. No two molecules of humus, completely broken-down soil, are or will ever be alike, like snowflakes or boy bands. Yes, it can be slightly messier than the surgical sterility of perlite or clay pellets, but if I have my way, earth underneath the fingernails will be a badge of honor in the near future.

> Sterilizing Soil at Home
>
> When using "found" soil and you're unsure about the benevolence of its community of microorganisms, sterilizing your soil will remove concern about mold growth or pathogens. Influence by unfriendly bacteria, molds, or fungus shouldn't be a major source of distress, as we're cutting the grass or green above the soil line and influence of these critters, but if you don't want a culture of fuzzy growth marring the beauty of your indoor garden, or you have pets or kids in the house, you may want to utilize one of these four methods to remove unknown factors from your soil.

Oven Method - Spread soil not more than four inches deep in non-plastic containers, such as seed flats, clay pots and glass, pyrex, or metal baking pans. Cover each container tightly with aluminum foil. Insert a meat or candy thermometer through one of the foil covers, and into the center of the soil. Set the oven between 180° and 200° F and watch the thermometer. Heat the soil to at least 180° F and keep it at this temperature for 30 minutes. Do not allow the temperature to go above 200° F - higher temperatures may produce plant toxins. Then cool, remove containers from the oven and leave the foil in place until ready to use. The heated soil will give off an odor somewhere between pungent earth and caramel.

Microwave Method –Microwave soil for 90 seconds per kilogram (2.2 pounds) on full power. Don't use metal containers and aluminum foil when using a microwave.

Use quart-sized plastic containers with lids, such as yogurt cups. Check the rims of the containers to make sure there is no aluminum of any kind; eradicate any trace of metal or foil seal. Fill the containers with very moist soil and cover. Poke a hole through the plastic lids with a nail for steam ventilation; a plastic temperature probe goes half way down into the soil through this hole in one of the containers. In a carousel-type microwave oven, heat the soil to 200°F and maintain that temperature for 20 minutes, varying the cooking program as necessary. In a large microwave, up to 7 quart containers can be sterilized at a time, making this a very efficient way to sterilize soil. Allow container to cool and put a piece of tape over the holes in the lids to keep the soil sterile until you're ready to use it.

You can also use a zip-loc gallon freezer bag; wet soil, leave the top open and place in the center of your carousel microwave. Treat for 2.5 minutes on full power (about 650 watts). After treatment allow the soil to cool and close the top of the bag.

Not a bad idea for cleaning soilless media in between hydroponic usages, which are susceptible to algal growth.

Steam Sterilization - Pour about an inch of water into a large pot. Fill containers that will fit in the pot (like loaf pans, baking pans, or glass canning jars) with leveled, loosely packed soil. Cover each container with aluminum foil. Stack the containers, if possible, to allow steam circulation. Leave the bottom container empty, or put the filled containers on something to keep them above the water. Cover the pot and bring the water to a boil. When steam begins to escape, continue boiling for 30 minutes at the lowest setting that will still produce steam. Turn off the heat and replace the lid. Remove soil when cool.

Make sure that your sterilization stays below 200° F – heavier soils and soils containing large amounts of organic matter may release compounds toxic to plants when heated too long or at too high a temperature. These toxins can cause poor seed germination or weakly plants. The toxicity is caused by an accumulation of ammonium compounds (see pee warning above), soluble organic compounds (the breakdown of which increases with heat, making the soil too rich for growing food), or high-temperature activation of salts. If there's a really convenient place for you to get you soil but it's yielding strange results, use a simple test to determine if the sterilized soil is toxic to plants: sow a few lettuce or other seeds with a high germination rate in both the treated and untreated soil and see what happens.

Because soil is only lacking in the easiness and cleanliness departments, I've devised a couple of techniques to make it just as easy to work with as the more futuristic and expensive options. The standard planting trays that are 20" by 10" take a little less than a gallon of dirt. Organic soil is available from nurseries and hardware stores in sizes starting at 8 quart bags, or 4 gallons. Take some gallon-sized zip-loc bags to the store with you, and in the parking lot, scoop the soil into 4 baggies (or however many you get out of the bag you bought.) Leave a little room in there; and keep it loose - if you pack it too tightly you'll end up with more than a trayful. Then go back in the store and throw the bag away in their garbage and wash your hands. Back home, you can store your bags in a plastic tote or an unused drawer in the kitchen, but if you're putting it somewhere that you don't want dirt, make sure you put it in a garbage or plastic grocery bag for safety. Then when you're ready to do some planting, dump the dirt into your tray, turning the bag inside out, and put your hand in the inside, formerly the outside (and more importantly the clean side), and use it like a mitten to smooth the dirt. Turn the bag right-side out and zip it (now the dirt is on the inside again and sealed), storing it for the next time you go to the store. Larger bags of soil are obviously cheaper than smaller, so if you have the storage, I recommend buying 40 lb. or 32 quart bags and filling up 7 or 8 gallon zip-locs per, respectively.

The second technique skips the bags and instead stores dirt directly inside a lidded plastic tub, which range in size from mouse coffin to garrison. They're sold at storage and discount stores, and are often available with wheels. They can be filled with soil and a plastic cup or scoop kept inside, the lid doubling as a work table when it's flipped over and laid across the top of the open bin perpendicularly. Very easy. Like most things in the book, these two techniques require a little bit of simple prep, but then actually doing them is a breeze.

Soilless Media

Several options are available if you don't want to deal with finding or using dirt. **Rock wool** is a combination of rock and sand, spun into matted fibers that are formed into many shapes and sizes. It's made in a similar way to cotton candy, and was originally used as wall insulation until its best virtues were discovered. It retains both moisture and air very well but is only usable once, and buying a new mat for every tray of grass at $4 or so, while still far cheaper than buying shots of wheatgrass at your local juice bar, is not the best option. Same goes for **baby blanket**, a thin organic pad sold in foot-wide rolls, **Tencel**, a eucalyptus-derived polymer, **coconut fiber**, a waste product of the coconut industry made from powdered husk, and **sphagnum**, a matted moss, and **peat moss**, which takes so long to grow that it's just not sustainable. **Coarse sand and clay**, if they're available to you, are good options for root support, though they will quickly dry out and don't hold nutrients for very long. Either one can add drainage to soil if your source is too dense and holds too much moisture. **Perlite** is a volcanic mineral that when heated to over 1600 degrees pops like popcorn and cools full of tiny air bubbles. The soft beads now resemble pearls, and have the unique ability to expand to 20 times their size when soaking up water. For this reason, they're an excellent addition to soilless growing mediums like sand that don't retain moisture well. Perlite is also pH-balanced, and can stabilize the acidity or alkalinity of the medium you choose.

Though the cost of soilless media is the main deterrent (with a consideration to the environmental impact of packaging, marketing, and shipping) most of them retain moisture for longer than dirt, which can be handy if you have less time to water or are going out of town for a few days. In an area of medium humidity, soil-based plants require watering about once a day at the beginning (with water needs increasing as the plants get bigger). If I'm going out-of-town for a few days to a week and don't want a lag in my grasses or greens, I'll start them in a moisture-retaining soilless medium like rock wool or coconut fiber, which I have for just this occasion, pre-soaked in fertilizer and water for a full day before they're planted. I'll leave 1/8" of the water sitting in the bottom of the tray for the medium to wick upwards as needed. I cover the tray with a clear greenhouse dome or plastic wrap and say a little prayer to the water gods. When I get back I'll give them a good watering, and I'm often pleased to return to hardy little plants, rebelliously growing happily without my care.

The above are materials commercially-labeled as soilless media, but anything that will hold moisture in and plants up will do. Ground Styrofoam packing peanuts, window screen, sea sponge; these and much more are viable options, depending on what's abundantly available to you.

Sprouts still have a rich food source to draw from, like an egg, but once they've doubled in size, they need to be given another source of food. Soilless media require fertilization, because unlike dirt, they don't have any of their own build-in minerals or soil-based organisms to continuously transform the plant's wastes into fresh, usable raw materials for healthy growth. More on this later, but keep in mind when choosing a medium that sowing a seed in the ground and keeping it moist is just *allowing* the earth to obey the inscrutable mandate of its nature, and create new life from old: the decaying plant and animal matter that makes up soil is transformed by an invisible microbial workforce into nutrients that feed adeptly sprouting seeds in millions of processes that science will never fully understand. Saying "this plant needs such and such nutrients to grow" sequesters a growing procedure from the mysterious and miraculous process that begot and continues life on Earth. Certainly, buying seeds online with paypal, having them shipped across the country, germinating them in a jar and spreading them in a tray in your windowsill isn't exactly a shamanistic approach to honoring the elemental forces that sustain life, but we do what we can. If it's growing wheatgrass in a Hello Kitty lunchbox under a reptile light you found in a dumpster or nothing, I'd obviously recommend the former. Just like a blade of grass can't be recreated in a lab, there are aspects to soil and plant nutrition that we don't understand and therefore can't duplicate artificially. So if you have a choice, and it's not so tedious or messy that it will keep you from your grass, natural, organic soil is best.

Containers

The standard receptacle for growing grass is a nursery tray, black or terra cotta-colored plastic rectangles about 20" by 10" by 2" deep with holes in the bottom for drainage. They're available online or in hardware, nursery or hydroponic stores for about $5 each. They are often sold alongside deeper trays that can catch drips, and high, domes clear plastic covers that retain moisture and turn the setup into a mini greenhouse. You only need 2 or 3 of these little kits, and in my opinion the price is low enough to curb more creative options. The shallow trays have thin channels running long ways along the floor of the container, and for some reason, the holes are always on the higher level of the bottom, in between the channels, allowing a good deal of water to sit in the tray. This can cause rot and mold. I recommend adding lots of holes to the lower-most surface of the tray by poking and twisting with a sharp, pointy knife, leaving an open circle that's big enough to let water drain out but small enough to keep dirt in.

Putting the 2" holed tray into a deeper tray not only collects the water that will continue drip out, it both allows for air circulation underneath your plants (important if you live in a tropical place or are growing in a humid season), and keeps moisture in for those that live in arid regions. Experiment with the clear cover, if you opt to use it, for moisture retention. It's also a visual indicator of moisture: you'll want to have a fine fog on the inside of the plastic; if the inner surface is dry there's not enough water, and if whole drops are collecting and running down the walls, it's too wet.

If you're getting the same kind of mold every time you grow, for example, a white fuzz that looks like fluffy cotton, you might want to try using the cover to protect your crop from airborne spores. Keep the clear cover over the plants anytime they're exposed to outside air. Remove the cover, water and drain it in a protected place, like your shower, then replace the cover before you put it back in the windowsill or outdoors. Mold isn't actually a big deal; just cut your grasses above the unwanted growth and rinse them before use. Sprouting and growing grasses is such a short-term endeavor that many pest problems that plague vegetable gardeners can be ignored or dealt with in a quick and superficial way.

There is no limit to what can be used as a growing container; if you don't want to spend the money for the prettily matching tray setup, you can use any vessel you have lying around. Cracked Tupperware containers, clay planter dishes, cookie sheets, the plastic clamshells that salad greens come in, old shallow bowls; anything that will hold dirt will do. If there aren't any drainage holes, you'll have to either punch some in the bottom (you can line it with coffee filters if your container comes pre-holed or cracked, or you were too enthusiastic with your hole-making) or you can just hold the growing medium and seeds in with your hands and tilt the container so that as much water as possible drains out. Many seasoned wheatgrass growers use trays with no drainage holes and use the tilt-drain technique; there's no shame in no holes.

Light

Plants require full spectrum, or "all color", light if they are to develop chlorophyll. Grasses grown without a good light source will be pale yellow, thin and sickly. There are two options: sunshine and artificial light. In the same way that modern science doesn't fully understand how microbes in dirt compost wastes into a myriad of nutrients, we have only a very basic knowledge of the effects of natural and artificial light on plant and animal growth.

Sunlight, when shined through a prism, will break up into the colors of the rainbow. This is the visible spectrum of electromagnetic energy, a tiny fraction of the wavelengths that make up light. Infrared (less than red) and ultraviolet (more than violet) light are the two wavelengths that bookend visible light and, though we can't see them, are essential to life. Infrared frequencies provide heat, without which life would be impossible, and ultraviolet light is responsible for chemical reactions such as those that help us create vitamin D, which helps us use calcium, regulate insulin, and power up our immune system.

Artificial light doesn't produce an even amount of each wavelength, but has peaks and valleys throughout. Sometimes this is the best that can be done with the type of bulb being used, and sometimes it's based on the manufacturer's preference. If you think you can choose the kind of light you use based on the amounts of each wavelength and your growing needs, consider this: when John Ott, of the Time Lapse Research Laboratory, studied the effects of artificial light on pumpkins in the mid-seventies, he found that the female pumpkin-producing flower withered and died under pinkish-white light, and consequently didn't produce fruit. When more blue was added to the spectrum to remedy this, the female buds produced bountifully while the male buds shriveled and fell off. In these artificial light conditions, reproduction could not take place.

Artificial light does just affect the different sexes of plants; the animal world is also adversely effected by variances from natural light. In an experiment conducted to see the effects of different kinds of light on animals, 1000 mice were divided into three groups, each with its own light environment. Those receiving natural daylight produced an equal amount of male and female offspring; those under white fluorescent bulbs produced 70% females and 30% males; and those under pink fluorescent bulbs produced 30% females and 70% males. For some reason we still don't understand, the latter group wasn't as healthy as either of the two other groups. All those exposed to the pink light quit breeding two months earlier and died one month earlier than those in the other groups. Humans are also affected by exposure to artificial light. In countries with long winter nights, it's been noticed that girl reach sexual maturity months or years younger than their grandmothers did. Assuming no change in diet or lifestyle (improbable, but it was their experiment, not mine. See pg 49 for effect of diet on hypermaturation), it was concluded that their normal rate of maturation is adversely affected by the introduction of artificial light.

The allure of artificial light is tempting, and appliance-like machines are available that can grow veggies and herbs from a dark corner with packets of plant vitamins and robotic precision. Under artificial light apples will grow larger than their natural counterparts, but will never ripen, a fact that's easy to miss when growing non-flowering, non-fruiting plants such as grasses or micro-lettuces. When choosing a spot for your grass, and all of the food in the next chapter that needs light to thrive, I strongly encourage you to seek out natural light, whether through a window, or on a porch or rooftop. If the eerie examples above inspire you set up a complex network of mirrors or knock on your neighbor's door with an offer to build a plant hammock or dumb waiter between your two apartments, then I've done my job, but if you've maximized your available natural light (quite easy to do in apartment and city-living), by all means supplement with artificial. I've just harped on the difference to curb lazy, unnecessary, and expensive glow-light set-ups. That, and it's fascinating.

Keep in mind that grasses don't need much direct light, and too much will burn and dry them out. Diffused or filtered light is best, for about 14 hours a day, though an hour or two of direct light and 8-10 hours of filtered light also produces good results. Experiment, and pay attention to the following factors: depth of green color (how much chlorophyll is being made), thickness of the blades (juiciness), and speed of growth (in the natural world, less light usually follows colder temperatures, and thinking it's winter the plants will grow more slowly).

If you've done all you can to pipe all of the available natural light onto your little patches of garden, artificial light may be necessary to supplement the sun or extend the day. When I lived in sunny Southern California, I was in a hilly, dense woods and only one window got any appreciable amount of outside light, which was indirect for most of the day. So I built shelves on that window (a rolling wire shelving unit would have worked just as well, but this place was so tiny that my shelves were made of clear Plexiglas and fold down when they're not in use), each of which has a T5 glow-light mounted to the bottom. The lights are daisy-chained together, and are moveable so that, if I was nearing harvest time on a flat of wheatgrass and it's a rainy day, I could move all 4 lights to one shelf. I moved my flats outside onto my stairs on the mornings that I'm home, but my grow-lights and timers, set from 7 AM to 9 PM, made it possible for me to enjoy fresh, nearly free wheatgrass juice every day. It also adds bright, full (visible) spectrum light to my apartment from the vicinity of the windows; not a bad thing. The shelves were packed up and went with me to Portland, where they're quite useful.

Fertilization - Feed Your Soil, Not Your Plants

We can't use the minerals in soil directly. To our metabolisms, they are just tiny rocks. We need a plant to uptake the nutrients and add an atom of carbon, thereby turning them into nutritious and delicious vitamins and minerals. In the same way, plants can't use nutrients directly from other plants and animals, which is why kitchen compost and animal wastes can't be added directly to the soil for instant plant food. It first has to be digested by microorganisms, who lovingly start the cycle over again.

A century of soil depletion has left our food nutritionally empty. Modern agriculture has discovered that plants need 3 nutrients to do the basic process of growing and bearing fruit: potassium, nitrogen, and phosphorous. There are over 100 minerals in healthy soil, and though different plants need different nutrients to be healthy, it's usually in the 50-100 range. With the 3 basic nutrients, plants are weak and sickly. They have no immune system of their own, and millions of tons of new pesticides are dumped on the world's farmlands every year. If it's not in the soil, it's not in the plant. These nutrient-deficient "foods" have no flavor - it's like eating a picture of a tomato – it may look like a tomato, but it doesn't taste like a tomato, nor (most importantly) does it nourish like one. Our grandparents can tell you what food tasted like before the mass depletion of nutrition from the soil. There are plenty of carbs in modern veggies, basically sugars linked together to form chains, but not much else. One of the greatest things about growing your own food is that you can increase the nutrients your plants are getting. If it's not in the plant, it's not in us, and by taking responsibility for what's in the soil, growing medium, and water (in the case of sprouting) of our Kitchen Sink Farms we can become want we want to be.

As mentioned above, when growing on soilless media it's necessary to fertilize your crops. Grass seeds will quickly use up the nutrients packaged into their hulls, and like a marooned spaceship will soon send out tiny probes in search of moisture and food. Even when growing in freshly composted, nutrient-rich soil, additional trace elements can only help. There are two types of fertilizers (we'll only be dealing with organic ones here, for what I hope by now are obvious reasons): those that are added to the germination and watering water, and those that are added to the growing medium. Though there are many options for each, I recommend only two for grass and micro-greens, and both are of the first variety. Grasses, as I've mentioned, are a relatively quick crop, and all the great nutrients in soil additives go largely unused. We'll come back to them when we discuss container gardening, but for now we'll stick to liquid fertilizing. Both liquid kelp fertilizer and ocean-based mineral solutions utilize the sea's inherently full spectrum of elements to provide your plants with all the nutrients they can use. Both are incredibly concentrated (dilute them with water 700:1 and 100:1, respectively) so one $15-$30 bottle lasts so long that it might just get passed down to your grandchildren. They're also really easy to use; just soak and water with the diluted solution like it's regular water. An easy and cheap source of nutrition, and you might want to leave it at that.

In the Kitchen Sink Farmer tradition, however, it is possible to make one's own fertilizer, traditionally called a "compost tea". A sprout bag or nylon stocking filled with a cup or two of blended compost is submerged in a gallon jar of water in a bucket. A teaspoon (1/2 oz) of unsulphured molasses is added to the brew as a food source for microorganisms. Cover it if gathering bugs will bother you, otherwise open is fine. In about 2 weeks you'll have your very own nutrient-rich and biologically-active compost tea, which will be diluted and added to your sprouting soak water and sprayed onto your plants; a light mist every day for grasses and microgreens, and a thorough watering once every week or two for container plants.

The same method can be used for "manure tea" if you have access to organically-fed livestock. "Hu-manure" can be processed in the very same way, and though we cringe at the thought in civilized society, I'm sure than future apartment farmers, who eat only pure, organic food full of healthy microorganisms, will appreciate the opportunity to live in a closed-system, creating no waste and being totally self-sustaining by resourcefully recycling everything.

H, P, and That Sneaky Little O: Hydrogen Peroxide

Another additive to consider is Hydrogen Peroxide, H_2O_2. As you can see from the chemical formula, Hydrogen Peroxide, or HP, is just water with an extra atom of oxygen. Oxygen is a very unstable element, and can be easily transferred from one molecule to another as it does in the upper atmosphere, where hydrogen gas (H_2) snags an oxygen or two from ozone (O_3), making both water and HP. Both will fall to the earth as rain, and the HP will keep its extra O unless it comes into the presence of a molecule with unstable atoms, like pollution, which will steal away the extra oxygen in an effort to stabilize itself. When HP can survive long enough to fall on plants, it adds extra oxygen to their life processes and neutralizes fungus and harmful bacteria in the soil.

The instability of oxygen is quite a lucky accident, because the beneficial bacteria in fermentation and digestion are aerobic, or oxygen-loving. "Bad" bacteria, with whom we don't have a symbiotic relationship and can make us sick if they overgrow, as well as fungi, molds, viruses, and cancer cells, are anaerobic – they can only survive in an oxygen-free environment. A single oxygen molecule, a beneficial free-radical, will separate from the HP molecule and destroy an anaerobic cell. This reaction can be seen if HP is poured onto a cut; the foaming, bubbling reaction is the oxygen splitting off from what is now non-reactive water (this isn't recommended for first aid, however, as some body tissues are anaerobic and will be damaged). HP both stimulates our crops' growth and targets harmful microorganism, leaving the good guys healthier than ever. Like sending poisoned pork to a concentration camp.

HP is also produced inside the body. Vitamin C fights infection by stimulating the production of HP, which fires off the extra oxygen to destroy the foreign cells. The probiotic cultures in our digestive systems produce HP to protect themselves (and us, consequently) from the growth of harmful yeast, fungus, and bacteria.

HP is essentially an oxygen supplement. Using it during the germination and growing of plants will help them stay disease-free, and can make them grow twice as fast. Just

drip some food-grade 30% or 35% solution into the soak water, and dilute it about 1 part HP to 10 parts water for watering. While you're at it, the same dilution ratio works great as a fruit and vegetable wash, facial toner, hand sanitizer, or kitchen and bathroom disinfecting cleaner. The solution can be added to baking soda for an old-school

---

Everyday Algebra

When using HP on the skin or in the mouth it's a good idea to be a bit more exacting with the 3% concentration. If 3% isn't available, or you buy 35% to save money or space, the dilution formula is Volume 1 times Concentration 1 = Volume 2 times Concentration 2, or $V_1(C_1)=V_2(C_2)$, with the concentrations being what you're starting (1) and ending with (2), and volumes being what you're trying to figure out (1) and what you want to end up with (2). It's actually really easy; use it once or twice and you'll have it down.

So if you're starting with 35% and want a liter of 3%, it's:

V1 times 35% = 1L times 3%

> V1 times 35 = 3
>
> (divide both sides by 35 – starting to ring a bell?
>
> V1 = 3 divided by 35
>
> V1 = .0085L, or 85mL (you could also start with V2 as 1000mL)
>
> In your liter jar pour in 85mL of 35% HP and fill the rest with water. Presto, you're a mathemagician. How you figure out 85mL is up to you (canning jars have 100mL marks on the sides, a kitchen scale is also handy, or use a dropper - about 10 drops equals 1mL.)

whitening toothpaste, and used full strength is a non-toxic laundry bleach or energizing bath additive, adding oxygen and scavenging bad bacteria wherever it goes. When I travel, I carry a 3.4oz (100mL, the maximum allowed in carry-on luggage) plastic dropper bottle of 35% HP and an empty spray bottle with a mark where it should be filled to. I can fill the spray bottle (with UV-sanitized water if I'm in a developing country) and use it for sanitizing my hands, toothbrush, dishes, toilet seats, ears after swimming, and anything else that has a ticket to my insides, as a facial toner and of course, sprouting accomplice.

Doin'It

Now that we've thoroughly covered the basics, we'll go over the actual recipe for growing wheatgrass and micro-lettuces like sunflower and pea.

Sprout 2 C. (8 oz) of seeds in the normal way. Remember that seeds with hulls, such as sunflower, will float, so they must be submerged or weighed down as described in the sprouting section. When the tails are about as long as the seed, they're ready to be planted.

Spread the growing medium in a tray, and pour the seeds evenly over the surface. There's no need to bury the seeds; the tails will root down and we'll keep them in the dark until they've got a solid foundation. Cover the seeds with a paper towel and water them thoroughly. The paper towel keeps the seeds from moving while they're watered and also block out the light so that they think they're underground – they won't be very enthusiastic about growing if they think they could be disturbed at any moment. Block out the rest of the light by covering the whole thing with a towel, or keep them in a dark place, such as a shower floor in a dark bathroom, closet, or a covered plastic storage container.

Keep them moist by spraying the paper towel a couple of times a day, and in a couple of days the roots that started when sprouting will spread and bury themselves, with little white points shooting straight up from the seeds. These are the infant grasses, and they're ready for the light. Put them under filtered sun, artificial light, or a combo of the two. It's quite remarkable how quickly they green up, and a new tray of grass is always a source of entertainment and wonder for this reason.

All that's left to do is water - one daily watering is enough if you live in a humid jungle, three may be necessary if you're in a bone-dry desert, but two waterings, in the morning and evening, is just right for most of us. I take my shallow dirt-filled trays out of their deeper drip trays, put them on the floor of my shower, and spray them thoroughly with my chlorine-filtering shower handle. After they drip fairly dry, I put them back in the drip trays.

When the grass is 6-8 inches high, it's at the peak of nutrition and ready to be harvested. I start cutting when the grass is about 4 inches so that by the time I reach the end of the tray it's no more than 8. If the grass is growing out of control, feel free to cut it all, put it in a zip-loc, suck out as much air as possible, and stick it in the fridge. It's better to use it freshly cut, though. To cut it, you can use clean scissors, holding a tuft of grass and snipping it just above the seed, or saw it off with a sharp or serrated knife.

Easy enough

How to Juice Grass

There are specific juicers just for wheatgrass that crush the grass by means of a turning screw. The dry pulp comes out one hole, and the bright green juice comes out another, right into your cup. They're powered by hand or electricity, and if you drink a lot of straight juice, one is probably a good investment (they start at $40 and go up to a couple of hundred). Grass juices can go from a sweetish just-mowed lawn flavor (wheat) to bitingly bitter and acrid (barley), so many people like to mix it with other flavors. I'm one of them, and I don't have room for a grass juicer, so I use my high-speed blender. Drop a large handful of freshly-cut grass into water, vegetable or apple juice, kombucha, kefir, or whatever you prefer, and blend the grass on high for 30-45 seconds. This will heat up the blender's contents, so some ice can be thrown in at the end if you like your juice cold. Ice can be water or fruit juice, by the way.

Your concoction is ready to drink, pulp and all, right out of the blender. If you wait a minute or two, though, all the pulp (indigestible fiber) will float to the top, and tilting the blender will pour out only the liquid, leaving the pulp behind. We all know the benefits of fiber for digestion and aging, but maybe just drinking a superfood that you grew yourself is enough right now.

If you don't have a wheatgrass juicer or high-speed blender, a regular juicer won't really do. All that yummy pulp will quickly gum up the screen and you'll be left with a wet mess. A regular blender or food processor isn't the best choice, but if that's all ya got, here's what you do. In the blender, pulverize the grass as much as possible; just beat it up like it stole your girlfriend. Then dump it into a sprout bag, clean panty hose, or other sieve-like fabric, and squeeze out as much juice as possible over a bowl. You won't get as much liquid this way than if you were to use a fancy machine, but it's a lot better than nothing. And if you know you're only going to get 2/3 the amount of juice out of a tray as your friends, plant another tray and you'll have 1/3 more than them. Now who's fancy?

My favorite grass in the wheat family is Kamut. It's never been hybridized or genetically modified like common wheat, has never seen a chemical pesticide or fertilizer, and its big fat seeds yield thick juicy grass. It's also a lot more nutritious than the common wheat all juice bars sell - another reason to grow your own. Spelt is my second choice (see "Kitchen Sink Farming Volume 1: Sprouting", Appendix A – Sprouting Seeds for more on kamut and spelt). Spelt is slightly more expensive than kamut and takes a few more pre-soak rinses to come out clean. It is, however, sweet and delicious, and far preferable to modern wheat.

Micro-Lettuces, Shoots and Greens

As I mentioned in the first paragraph of this section, any leafy green sprout can be grown into a micro lettuce or micro green. It's as simple as sowing your seeds into a soil or soilless medium-filled tray and keeping it moist. The

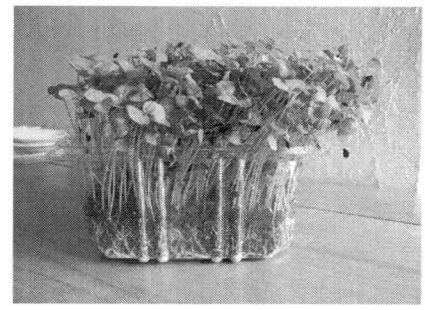

Watercress micro lettuce

process is the same as grasses, though the germination (soaking and sprouting) phase happens right in the dirt. Seeds grown into micro lettuces are always quite small, so soaking is a cinch – your wet paper towel will keep the seed buried and moist, so that's all there is to it. Also, microgreens are much less light sensitive; just 3-6 hours of diffused sunlight is plenty, though pale and leggy plants grown in a lightless bookshelf wouldn't be the end of the world. This is also a great first-dirt project, because you'll only have to keep them alive for a couple of weeks, tops.

Choosing your plants

Each micro-lettuce will grow at a different speed in different conditions. Some greens are ready in 1 week, while others can take 3 weeks. For this reason, I recommend starting out with mono-crops, planting for example, a tray with arugula, one with alfalfa, and one with broccoli, and as some grow quickly and some take their sweet time, you'll always be in the micro-greens. The other option is to use an organic micro-greens mix, which has been put together to compliment taste and growing time. It's also a good way to try things you wouldn't (or can't) buy and plant separately, like Cherry Belle Radish, Beet Bulls Blood , Pak Choy, Cabbage Red Ace, Kohlrabi , Swiss Chard Lucullus, and others, commonly found in mixes but pretty much impossible to find on their own. Seed packets are also quite inexpensive at $2-3, and because we're growing them past the sprout stage a little goes a long, long way.

It should be no surprise by now that my favorite option is to DIY and make my own mix. After you can identify individual varieties of micro-lettuces and combine them in appetizing ways, it's quite easy to buy a few grams of each and sow 'til your heart's content. I'm slowly discovering mild, tangy, Provencal, and Asian mixes that suit my palate. I buy the organic seed packets and dump them all together into a small, dry bottle, ready to be sprinkled onto a fresh bed of dirt.

Week-old cilantro micro-lettuce

The last step in sustainability in micro lettuces is to harvest your own seeds. This would mean growing a few micro-lettuces into a larger container, and letting them go to seed; collecting, drying, and saving the seeds for future plantings. Buying packets of organic seeds online or at the local natural foods store is a luxury and in the event of a disaster, natural or otherwise, the person who is already living in a self-sufficient manner is going to be eating much better than those that have to scramble to get set up.

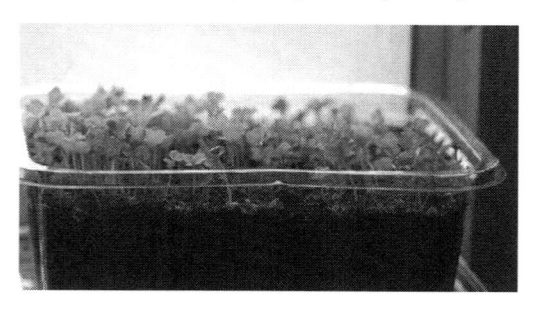

Another important difference between growing micro-lettuces and grasses is that the lettuce won't mat the soil with a resolute root system, allowing most of the growing medium to be used again. For this reason, it's fine to plant in a deeper container, pulling out the roots of your last harvest and tilling the soil (that means turning it over to mix the nutrients, for you city folk) with a fork. Deeper containers include plastic clamshells that spinach and herbs are sold in and restaurant Styrofoam to-go containers. Punch ¼" holes in the bottom every 4-5 inches, and use the lid of the container as a drip tray. Fill it with soil, leaving ½" of space at the top so that watering doesn't overflow the container, and moisten well. Sprinkle your seeds on the soil and cover with a paper towel or 1/8" more dirt, and spray that with a little water to get them germinating.

Keep the top layer of soil moist but not wet. When the sprouts start pushing up the paper towel, remove it and put the container in the sunniest window you've got. The micro-lettuces can be harvested after a week or two; the best time is right before the second set of leaves opens. The first leaves are called "seed leaves", and the second "true leaves", and when these come about the plants gets ready for the long haul, trading in tender deliciousness for increased nitrogen uptake, causing a tougher texture and more bitter flavor. Unlike grass, the cut lettuces won't grow again, because they're still technically sprouts.

Start a new batch when your current crop is a week in, and you'll have micro-lettuce salads all year round.

Shoots

Larger seeds such as legumes and shell-on sunflower can be grown into larger veggies. Like grains grown into grasses, they must first be soaked and sprouted a little before they're sown on a growing medium, which allows them to be germinated evenly without having to be sown underground, bringing up the dirty dirt with them as the grow. The seed will rest on top the dirt, the root will go down, and the clean stalk and leaves will go the opposite direction. A legume will quickly shoot up a tall, straight stalk, and small leaves will begin to develop when it's 3 or 4 inches tall. This is called a "shoot", and should be harvested soon after the first pair of leaves open, or it can get tough. If the second set of leaves open before you can

cut them, they will be
quite un-chewable, and
their best use is one that
utilizes the high-speed
blender.

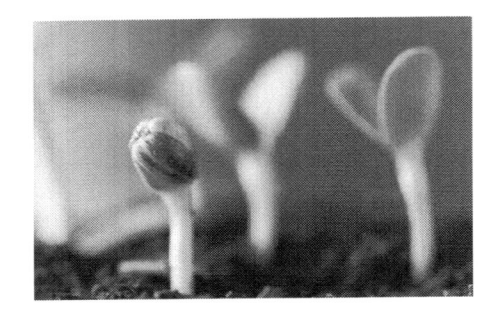

Sunflower Lettuce

One of my favorite greens, sunflower lettuce is cheap and easy to grow into thick and crunchy double-leafed tendrils. They are cultivated the same way as grasses and legumes, but their deliciousness deserves a special mention. Also, their shells require a slightly different technique during both soaking and harvesting.

Sunflower seeds in the shell will float,

Sunflower micro-lettuce

staying dry, if left to their own devices. Put them in a jar with a screw-on lid and fill with clean water. The seeds will stay on top of the water as the level rises. Continue filling until the seeds are above the lid but not quite falling out, then screw a lid on to push the seeds down into the water, submerging them completely If there's still an air bubble, just shake the jar a couple of times during the soaking to rotate the dry seeds. . If you don't have a canning jar, they can be imprisoned in a sprouting bag and held down by rock in any water-filled container. Then sprout them for a day or so until a little turtle tail pokes out of the shell, and spread them on some dirt or other growing medium.

The other thing that's unique to sunflower lettuce is that the shell won't stay earthbound, but will slither upwards on top of the sprout, protecting the leaves until they're ready to come out. In 5-8 days the shells will begin dropping off as the pair of succulent green leaves swell and spread. It's great fun to listen to the seedpod dropping to the shelf or ground; it's how I imagine a jungle to sound. I like to eat them as soon as possible after this rite of passage. It feels, nutritionally speaking, that with luminous vitality they've shed their adolescence and are straightening themselves with a new and fresh adulthood, and stepping into the sunshine with their faces deliciously raised. That's when I bite down. Hey, it's a cruel world.

They can also be gently pulled off by hand. Notice the difference between leaves that were forced into maturity and those that came into it on their own. Try to do it with one hand without pulling the root up, and you've got yourself a game more fun than Operation, and with a much better prize at the end. Sunflower micro-lettuce is great wherever sprouts are used: sandwiches, warps and burritos, as a garnish for soups, in veggie juice and salads. In fact, sunflower greens have such a mild, crunchy, and fresh flavor that they can be the only lettuce in a salad, either kept whole or chopped.

Container Gardening

Outdoor Growing

It's quite feasible to grow herbs, any vegetable, even tree fruit like citrus, pears and apples from a small city apartment amongst sirens and smog. With attention to water, fertilization, light, and warmth, any balcony or landing can be made into a lush growing area that can feed you and your family or friends daily. On the 3 ½ foot square landing at the top of my stairs I'm growing 3 kinds of peppers, tomatoes, mint, 3 kinds of basil, tarragon, peas, and strawberries. I also have a large Meyer lemon tree that supplies me with a lemon or two per week, year-round, and months of the most heavenly scent imaginable. Container gardening can afford more flexibility than a traditional garden: move pots to follow the sun, bring them inside on frosty nights, or hang pots or bags above the tongues of hungry wildlife. It's also a good way to recycle containers and use found vessels: buckets, lined baskets, bathtubs, and vintage high-heeled shoes will all hold dirt, and therefore the roots of food. Just make sure they have a hole or holes for drainage.

Dirt and soilless media was covered at length in the last section, and all of that info holds here as well, with a thought towards longer-term plant needs. While the dirt used for a week of growing grass is quickly composted and forgotten, the growing medium that will nourish and sustain your plant and you for months or years requires a sustained-release nutritional support. Dirt purloined from a garden or park won't drain quickly enough for a container, so a soil mix is necessary. Your plants need a mix that holds some moisture, but drains well, and contains a generous supply of nutrients to get the crop started off right. Though different types of plants have different moisture and nutrient needs, a good basic potting soil is one part dirt from the ground, one part sand, and one part composted soil or worm castings. If you live in an arid climate, less sand may be necessary; the opposite is true if your local earth has a lot of clay. A handful of perlite (see pg XX) will retain just the right amount of moisture, lighten the soil further, and help neutralize the pH. We'll need to re-fertilize at intervals – more on this a little later.

Light

This is the first thing that must be considered when planning your garden. It's a good idea to map out your space by the amount of sunlight each area gets. Small city spaces can have widely varying amounts of light in sections of rooms right next to each other, from several hours of full sun to only sparsely reflected light. When looking at your space this way, it's easy to start seeing the amount of food that can come from even the shadiest windowsill and teeniest patio.

Full Sun

If you're lucky enough to have a large window or patio with full sun, you'll have no problem growing fruit trees, berries, and all kinds of vegetables. Fruit, including fruiting vegetable such as bell peppers, eggplant, tomatoes, cucumbers, etc. need 4-5 hours of full sun a day, preferably more, and a few more hours of indirect or reflected light. Your main concern will be lack of space, and you'll have to consider temperature and humidity, but sun is usually the scarcest resource for most urban apartment dwellers so it's best to make the most of what full sun you have. If you have an outdoor area with plenty of light, I recommend focusing your container gardening efforts here, and once this space is maximized, branching out to the other possible growing areas in your home, office, and neighbor's places.

Medium Light

Plants that require less light energy are those with smaller fruit, like cherry tomatoes and chili peppers. Squash is easy to grow, but its size can be prohibitive in containers. Try a smaller variety like zucchini, which is even more versatile in the kitchen as it is the garden. Slower-growing varieties of legumes, such as bush peas and bush beans, require less sun than their more common counterparts, the "pole" varieties, which ultimately produce larger crops over time, and are a better choice if you have the light.

Possibly the most efficient use of medium light conditions is to grow plants for their seeds. Amaranth and quinoa, for example, produce huge clusters of nutrient-packed tiny seeds, which can be collected and sprouted for a very large amount of actual food from one plant, much more than can be harvested in fruit or vegetable mass.

Low light

The last place to spend your gardening energy can still be a very effective growing space. Root vegetables like beets, turnips, potatoes, and carrots can do very well with only a few hours of reflected light. Root and tuber plants are quite cooperative with Kitchen Sink Farming by storing most of their energy underground in the part that we harvest for food, so it's less important how much light they receive daily and more important how much sun they soak up over the entire season. Therefore, letting them go as long as possible before harvest will yield the fullest, juiciest roots. But all root vegetables can be harvested and eaten small, so even scraggly plants grown in paltry light can produce a delightful crop of baby root vegetables.

Lastly, leafy greens have fairly low light requirements than plants that we want for their flowers or fruit. Full sunlight may actually burn many plants that have evolved large, wrinkled satellite dishes for collecting scant illumination. They can be grown year-round in many climates, and many varieties can even be started in the fall for continuous winter salads. Beet and turnip greens, lettuces, kale, collard greens, arugula and spinach can also be defensively started inside, in front of a window or under a glow light then placed outside when they're a little more established. For the same reason, many ground-covering herbs like mint, rosemary, and tarragon can thrive in low light conditions.

Garlic is a quick-growing low light plant, whose shoots (chives) are just as delicious as the bulb-roots themselves. Stick a clove or two, point down, in dirt-filled plastic containers like yogurt cups and put them anywhere you want. Garlic will make the soil unusable by other plants so it's best grown alone, its bedding composted after the roots are harvested. Even the tiniest apartment will have more room for garlic than the tenant has appetite. Same goes for green or spring onions, which can go from ghostly white to deep purple in color, and pungent to sweet in flavor, so much so that some varieties are delicious eaten washed and raw. I made many meals of the wild onions that grew on the banks of the large river by my childhood Ohio home, cursorily cleaned in the swirling rapids. Today, a spring onion or two goes in just about every dressing and soup, providing the perfect multi-cylinder sharpness and fresh bite.

Maximizing Sun

If you're lucky enough to have no buildings blocking out the sun for some of the day, you'll want to think in three dimensions to maximize your amount of sun-sweet, chlorophyll-rich food. Terracing and vertical gardening are ways to keep plants from blocking each other and maximize precious floor space. Put taller trees, trellised vines, and peas, beans and corn closest to your wall, leaving a few inches for light to reflect onto the backs of the plants. You may also cover the wall with used aluminum foil, those silver tanning blankets people lay on at the beach for the same reason, reflective car sun shades, thermal emergency blankets, or anything else that will maximize your light in an otherwise unexpected direction. Medium height plants such as broccoli, cabbage, cauliflower, cucumbers, and tomatoes come next, with shorter plants like herbs and flowers in the front row. Arranging crops by height is called terracing, and is a simple technique used with great benefit for thousands of years in hilly farmland. If your crops aren't widely divergent in height, you can produce this effect by making steps, whether by building them out of scraps of plywood to fit your space, or stacking crates or plastic boxes to create the same result.

Now comes 3D-thinking to maximize space in the vertical axis: upside-down growing. This technique allows the ceiling of a patio to be used almost as efficiently as the floor. Baskets and bags are hung from hooks in the ceiling along with tumbling vines of tomatoes, peppers, strawberries, herbs, or baby vegetables like patty pan squash or Persian cucumbers. Not as pretty than wire baskets or store-bought grow bags, but possibly more effective because of their dark, sun-sucking color, are diy grow bags made with those reusable grocery totes with doubled plastic grocery bags or plastic trash can liners on the inside. A few well-placed horizontal slits on the front surface of the totes (put a cutting board inside the bag and cut the tote and liners at the same time with a utility knife) will make pockets for your berries or baby zucchini to be planted in. Fill the bag half full with potting soil, place the roots of your seedlings in through the slits, and after seeing if its handles need to be reinforced, hang it from a strong hook screwed into a joist (2x4 running underneath the surface of the ceiling. Find them, and learn which direction they run, with a stud finder or by knocking with your knuckles and listening for a higher-pitched, solider sound than the surrounding area). The color of tote or bag is an important consideration; darker will absorb as much warmth as possible, great for starting seeds and cooler months, but will require more water during warmer seasons, possibly 2 or even 3 times a day at the height of summer. Potting mixes are generally lighter than soil and are recommended to keep the bag from being too heavy. If your bags hang over a walkway or sitting area, make sure to check the integrity of the bag more frequently and diligently.

Plastic bags, especially the larger-sized, thick black liners can also be used instead of pots by simply poking some drainage holes and filling with soil and a single plant, or using the slit-pocket method described above. They can expand or shrink depending on the season by regulating the amount of dirt inside, and are (unfortunately for landfills) surprisingly durable. They can also be closed with a twist tie and laid on their sides, with slits cut into what is now the top and like a low, wide, flexible pot. This makes for a compact and easily moveable garden, if a sunny space is being used temporarily or without implicit permission. Plants can also be grown this way in a hammock slung between two balconies or posts.

PVC piping can also be used as an effective and versatile growing device. Drill or cut holes at least 1 ½" wide all around a length of PVC tubing, scraps of which are always available for free at lumber yards. There's also a pocket-cutting technique described in the "Growing Wall" section that's even better. You'll need to buy the right-sized cap for the bottom, and a chain or strong rope to attach to the top for hanging. Drill lots of small holes in the bottom cap and attach it to the pipe; you may want to glue it in place if the fit isn't snug, as it will be holding a lot of the weight of the soil and plants. Drill two more holes at the top of the tube to feed the chain, wire, or rope through (this will be getting wet so a synthetic, waterproof material is best) and hang it from a sturdy hook, preferably attached to a ceiling joist or other structural beam (see 2 paragraphs up). The end a hose can be left in the top to be turned on for a minute or two every day. If you have a spigot, setting up a drip system on a timer may be the best option for multiple hanging tubes, and the whole system can be made in an afternoon, the rest of a gardener's time free for sipping fresh strawberry margaritas and reading my blog (but if you're considering this set-up, check out the "Growing Wall" plans first).

Choosing Crops

When deciding what to grow, you have two options when conforming to the natural laws of space, light, warmth, etc. You can choose to grow a variety of fruits and vegetables, giving you and your family and friends varied nutrients and flavors. You can also grow a larger amount of fewer kinds of plants – finding the type and variety of plants that will net you that maximum food for your space. The latter route has two benefits. The first is that it will take less time, both in learning the different needs of your diverse garden and in tending. Much quicker to water everything at once, feeding all simultaneously with the same fertilizer, and dealing with pests with the single Hammer of Judah instead of the many pebbles of David. As most Kitchen Sink Farming projects are limited not by space but by time this can be a very big difference.

If you live away from people, or at least like-minded people, growing a myriad of different plants may be the way to go, but trading bushels of beautiful tomatoes for future vegetables of a different sort, or honey, milk, or anything else one person might have an abundance of, including services, is the best description of community I can think of. There's an African proverb that asks how someone can eat a fish for a year – the answer is that they divide it amongst their neighbors, who then share their food.

I started a non-profit in Portland called GardenAngels.org which turns the excess organic produce from overgrown gardens and public domain trees into non-perishable, raw foods like zucchini breads, fermented apple butter, and kale crackers, and distributes them to the needy. The gardener is repaid with prepared foods unless they'd like to donate their portion. Again, hunger is not a supply problem, it's one of distribution, as LA's sidewalks strewn with rotting oranges and downtown littered with hungry people attests to.

Indoor Growing

Many plants will do much better in indoor containers, a boon for the average urbanite who has much more indoor space than out. The inside of a window allows light that's almost as good to stream in to a temperature-controlled environment, and options for trapping heat and humidity abound. Some plants, like gingerroot, do better indoors, where the tropical conditions in which it thrives are recreated more easily than outside. Clear or wire shelving units (see my example on pg XX) are essential for growing grasses and micro-lettuces, and if there's still room, leaf and small-fruit plants than can utilize a slightly less powerful light should take up residence.

Self-Watering Containers

This simple and cheap development in container gardening is so easy to make and use it's just amazing that they're such a recent development. The advantages are several. They assure proper soil moisture at all times, eliminating thirsty plants, but also taking care of problems from over-watering, which can also starve the plants of precious oxygen or dehydrate them, as roots can't take in water when the soil's moisture is over 40%. Soil that's too wet can also contribute to many diseases such as root rot and mold. The layer of air at the bottom of self-watering containers increases oxygen to the roots of the plants, which breathe just like we do. They also strengthen the root system by inspiring them to reach down to get at the water, the way plants in nature grow, while top-fertilizing stimulates a second system of roots more toward the surface of the soil. This double-layer root system creates faster-growing and higher-yielding plants, which can often out-produce plants grown in the ground. The most important argument for self-watering containers, however, is that by essentially watering themselves from a back-up reservoir, you may be able to cut your container gardening efforts to once a week, freeing up time for other things. Not many farmers can go to Cancun in the middle of a growing season.

The underlying idea behind self-watering is a reservoir of water with a "wick" that draws moisture up into the soil. There are a few ways to do this, and after the couple of examples that follow the resourceful Kitchen Sink Famer will be able to easily create custom containers to suit their own purposes.

Simple Self-Watering Devices: "the spike" and "the holey bottle"

The Watering Spike

You'll need:

A 2-liter plastic bottle and a foot long piece of PVC that's slightly larger than the mouth of the bottle

Cut the bottom of the PVC at an angle, and drill holes in the sides, the size of which will be determined by the plants' water needs. Fill the 2 liter bottle with water and turn it over onto the PVC. This allows not only for the soil to regulate its own moisture level, but for the water to be delivered directly to the plant's roots. The spike will fill with soil when inserted, so it doesn't water as heavily as it would seem.

A plastic soda or water bottle can also be buried in the soil and filled with water; the size of the holes poked around the bottom of the bottle will determine the speed of flow.

The Self-Watering Bucket

Step One: Assemble your materials

These are:

A bucket,

A soil barrier,

Fabric wicks,

A watering tube,

A utility knife,

And soil.

Bucket – this could be a five gallon bucket and lid, or any two buckets that fit inside of each other, available from hardware stores, restaurants, nurseries, recycling centers, and many other places for cheap or free. Be careful not to use a bucket that's had paint or any other chemical in it, which will almost certainly end up in your soil, plant, food, and liver. My top choice is soy sauce buckets from Japanese restaurants for their cool labels, though many foods are packaged this way. You can also use a pretty plastic pot, or even a terra cotta one, for a more presentable planter. Any big enough container with no holes will do.

Soil barrier – something round that's small enough to slide inside the bucket but too big to go all the way to the bottom. If using a 5-gallon bucket, this can be the middle of the lid, cut out for this purpose (save the outer ring for step 3), a plastic planter tray, or an entire other bucket, if the bottoms are 4 far enough apart to leave room for the water reservoir. Make sure you can cut or drill holes in whatever you choose in the soil barrier. If the soil barrier doesn't leave enough room between the two (think 3+ inches, more if you want a bigger reservoir and less frequent refilling), a rock or block of wood can be put in to hold the bucket up higher. If you're using a tray-type soil barrier, make sure that there's still a tight fit around the edges because we can't let dirt fall through gaps into the water. The soil barrier will need to be stiff and strong enough to hold up the weight of the soil and plants.

Fabric wicks – We'll use a few foot-long, 1-inch-wide strips of cotton cloth; an old towel works well. The basket-wick described in the next plan uses soil to bring up water. This system requires a little bit more work but is also more effective.

Watering tube – This is how we'll fill the reservoir, bypassing the soil. The rigid tube needs to be a few inches taller than the bucket, and can be PVC pipe, plastic (including clear for sneakiness), bamboo or metal (like copper water pipe, cheap and lovely), depending on availability, cost, and aesthetics. I have faith in you.

Step Two: Cuts and Holes

1 - Place your soil barrier into your bucket, and drill or cut a few small holes about an inch above the bottom of the soil line around the side of your bucket. It's easier to do this from the inside of the bucket with the barrier in place. Sounds obvious, but I've seen plans that include complex ways for finding out where on the outside to drill. These holes allow oxygen in to the roots, creating faster-growing, hyper-producing plants, and btw this 30-second procedure should be done to all growing containers. Cut a larger (1/4" or so) hole an inch below the soil line; this will be the overflow hole to let you know the reservoir is full. If you're using a terra cotta or clay container (again, no holes at the

bottom) use a ¼" glass and tile drill bit, sprinkling water over it as you drill to keep it cool.

2 - Cut 3 small holes in the soil barrier, just big enough to pull the fabric wicks through.

3 - Cut a larger hole at the edge of the soil barrier, just big enough to fit the watering tube into. If it's not a really snug fit, cover the hole with a round piece of burlap or other coarse, thick fabric that's much bigger than it, and cut a small "X" in it for the tube to go into to keep soil from falling into the reservoir.

4 - Cut the bottom of the watering tube at an angle to allow a free flow of water when it sits on the bottom of the bucket or pot.

Step Three: Assemble your planter

Tie large, loose knots in the middle of your fabric wicks. Insert the wicks through the top of the holes in the soil barrier, until they reach the knots. Slide the soil barrier into the bucket, pushing down evenly on the edges until it's flat. Insert the watering tube into its hole and fill the bucket with pre-moistened, un-fertilized soil, leaving a couple of inches of room at the top.

If you'd like to use a moisture barrier, lay it over the top of the soil and attach the remaining outer ring of the lid, assuming you cut out the inside for your soil barrier. If you don't have a lid, tape works. A black plastic garbage bag is fine, though many other products are available. Cut X's in the barrier and insert your plants. Fill the reservoir with the watering tube, stopping when your overflow hole goes into action. Top fertilize every two weeks. Then hit travelocity.

The Self-Watering Garden

This is a larger-scale project, because it's hard to grow much food in a 5-gallon bucket. The concept is exactly the same (not repeated here so read the above first), but the details are a little more conducive to food growing. A large plastic tote, discarded bathtub basin, or kiddie pool are all perfectly acceptable containers, and again, having two of them that fit inside each other will make the process much easier. Otherwise, the lid is the next best option for a soil barrier, the edge cut off to form a tight fit and saved to hold down a moisture barrier, even more helpful with all the soil surface area you're about to have. You can also use two large plastic garbage bags with a rigid flat surface or lattice, and blocks or bricks to hold the inner one up. The watering tube is the same, but depending on the size of your garden you may want to use several, and you also might want to secure them to the sides of the container with a hot glue gun, bailing wire, duct tape, or a bolt. As mentioned above, the wick is going to be slightly more complicated, but also much better at distributing water evenly through soil, because the wick itself is made of soil.

The soil wick, or foot, is a plastic kitchen strainer, a "fish and chips" basket that seafood and sandwiches are sometimes served in, or a plastic bowl, small plastic planter, or other short fat container, with enough holes poked in it to resemble a basket.

If you're sticking with the 5-gallon bucket container because of its size and easy transportability, you may want to use a soil wick as well. Find a yogurt cup or similarly-shaped container and poke several dozen holes all around it. Pack it tightly with moistened soil and insert it into a hole cut in the soil barrier, small enough that it doesn't go all the way through.

Fertilizing

Non-organic fertilizers promise massive bright red tomatoes and watermelons the size of Volkswagens, but their allure quickly fades when you take of bite of the tasteless fruit. Organic fertilizers are tremendously more effective, better for everyone, and nearly free if you make them yourself. Every two weeks or so (more when your plants are producing), top-fertilize by adding compost tea to water and pouring it evenly over the dirt, or adding worm castings or freshly composted soil to the top of the soil and pouring some water over it to mix it up.

See "Plant Nutritional Deficiencies" on pg XX for specific nutrients needed by less-than-vibrant plants and where to get them.

Furthermore

Aside from light, dirt, fert, and water, the only thing left to discuss on the subject of growing food in a container is the stalk-by-stalk specifics of each plant's need. And this is probably the most important. Which is why I'm going to skip it.

There are piles of wonderful books, blogs, and local experts about your specific climate and what you want to eat, and I couldn't possibly cover it all here. So I'm going to leave it up to you to educate yourself, suggesting you start with one plant, maybe a citrus tree if you have a warm sunny spot, an herb or two if not, and think of them as houseplants 2.0. Add a plant or two to your patio or windowsill farm whenever you've gotten the hang of the last ones.

Hooked on 'Ponics: Hydroponic and Aeroponic Gardening

Sprouts grow quickly and, drawing nutrients from water, can increase 30 times in size. Next, we have micro-lettuces, that with a little bit of dirt can do even better. But if you want to grow a large amount of food, whether for your family or neighborhood to eat, barter, or sell, you'll need to know about hydroponics (from the Greek "to labor with water"). You've probably heard about hydroponics, a system that floods plants' roots with a nutrient-rich water solution, and aeroponics, which suspends plants' roots in an environment made humid and delicious by constantly or intermittently spraying them with a nutrient-water solution. Both have their benefits and drawbacks, and this section will go into more detail about their differences so you can make an informed decision about which is best for you.

Hydroponics and aeroponics are based on the fact that dirt serves only two functions – to hold the plant up and supply it with water and nutrients. Both hydro- and aero- grow plants without soil, which are held up by a soilless medium and fed with nutrient-rich water. The main difference is how that solution is fed – hydroponics washes the roots with a flowing current of water while aeroponics keeps the roots hanging in a constantly misty environment and sprays them with nutrients. Aeroponics is thought to be superior for several reasons, but hydro does have two advantages.

First: The Similarities

Plants grow much more quickly and produce more in a hydro or aeroponics set-up, because they're being spoon-fed readily usable nutrients; instead of having to spend energy growing roots and digesting what they find. They can put all of their effort into producing food. Because of this lack of hardship, their fruit isn't going to be as hearty and full of flavor as food grown in containers or the ground, but again, there's going to be a lot more of it. Also, because the roots aren't inspired to grow very long the pots stay small and closer together, making the system more compact than container or ground growing. But because the kinds of nutrients the plants are given directly affects the stage of growth they can enter - fruiting, flowering, seeding – the timing of all of these stages can be regulated. This means that if you're growing basil, which is an annual and seeds and dies at the end of the year, you can stick to the vegetative nutrients and stay in the pesto indefinitely. You can also grow, for example, a few amaranth or quinoa plants, which produce huge amounts of seeds, and keep them in the seed-production business just to have seeds to sprout to large quantities, potentially the most effective growing setup for feeding large numbers of people. I believe that having hydroponic "seed factories", then sprouting those seeds, both with home-made liquid fertilizer, to yield potentially thousands of times the amount of food that can be produced by growing a plant in a pot, will be the large-scale urban farming of the future, capable of feeding entire apartment buildings from the roof with an unending chain of week-long growing seasons, or the answer to the distribution issue of global hunger. Enough food can be produced to feed everyone in the world, many times more if we were all to become vegetarians. But the difficulty in *getting* the food to the people that need it is what keeps them hungry. "Sprouting seed factories" can be localized and many, and could be an answer.

Hydroponics and aeroponics are both beneficial to the environment because their carefully controlled growing environment makes chemical fertilizers and pesticides completely unnecessary. They both use less water and fertilizer than in-the-ground gardening, take up much less space (especially with the growing wall and bucket systems discussed later), and can be used anywhere, from underground basements and caves to space stations.

Now: the Differences

Of the two, aeroponics will yield about 25% faster results because the roots aren't suspended in water, and are therefore have access to more air. Plants' roots need oxygen to absorb nutrients, and carbon dioxide is a necessary factor in photosynthesis, another way plants feed. Hydroponics uses a mineral solution that can become infected with algae, parasites, and bacteria over the two-week period it's used. In aeroponics, the infestation of plants is minimized because each 15-minutes-apart nutrient spray is fresh and sterile. Contact between plants is also minimal in aeroponics, thereby preventing the spread of diseases. In aeroponics, gardeners have greater control over the growing environment, and properly maintained plants will be totally free from diseases and pests, while hydroponics cannot be so precisely controlled.

Aeroponics another edge in that it uses less water and only a quarter of the nutrient supply. It does require more electricity, however, because the pump that powers the misters is constantly going, as opposed to intermittent pumping in hydro. And because aeroponics is such a finely-tuned system, the result of a power failure is catastrophic; the plants will begin to wilt and starve immediately if the power goes out or more than one or two sprayers get clogged. For this reason, aeroponics requires more attention than hydro, which once established, can be left on its own for days or weeks. Many aeroponics growers that depend on the food they grow actually have a back-up hydro system in case of power failure.

Because there's a fairly constant water level in an aeroponics system, some people raise edible fish in the reservoir, which will raise the heat in the system (better for the plants) and fertilize the water. This called "aquiponics", and can be a completely self-enclosed system, with fish waste feeding the plants, the plants filtering out the waste (which is toxic to the fish), and algal growth feeding the fish. It's possible make an aquiponic set-up with the fill-and-drain of hydroponics, but the reservoir would have to be really big to keep the fish happy.

So when choosing between hydro and aeroponics to feed your family or community, it really comes down to two things: electricity and attention. A vacation home or remote greenhouse in an area with high-priced power or a just few solar panels? Hydro it is. A community garden or teen center with many hands and eyes and an abundance of free energy from wind, sun, or hydroelectric sources? Free to be aero. Your situation is most likely somewhere in between these two extremes, so your decision won't be quite so cut and dry. The good news is that both systems require the same amount of skill to build (e.g. – not very much) and will allow you to pretty much grow as much food as you want, being more limited by your time and passion than by your space and funds.

The Plans: Hydroponics

Hydro has one more advantage that wasn't mentioned earlier, the ability to build a system out of just about anything. While aeroponics can be conceivably carried out with a spray bottle and a whole lot of free time, it's a finely-tuned system that needs to be set up in a conscious way. Hydro, however, can be pretty much be slapped together from trash, and though it always incorporates a pump to flood the system, one could potentially just dump fertilized water over the plants' suspended roots a few times a day, collecting it as it drains, forego all fanciness and call it hydroponics. Conversely, to make a well thought-out and efficient system only requires a small pump ($5) and plastic tubing ($1.50), and it's quite possible to build the rest entirely out of found objects – discarded plastic tubs, 2 liter soda bottles from the recycling center, roadside gravel as a growing medium, etc. This section will teach you how to make compact, efficient, and automated systems that can be left alone for weeks at a time, customizable for your space, lighting requirement, handiness, and number of plants, and money-saving variations will be left up to your imagination.

But first, a note about algae:

Algae - which can be green, red, or brown - are a form of plant life that is a natural consequence of exposing nutrient-rich water to light. Algae aren't given a second thought by container growers but it can be a concern in hydroponic set-ups. They're actually non-toxic to your plants and can even supply extra nutrients, but as they bloom, die, and decompose they will rob your plants of valuable oxygen. They can also propagate on roots, limiting or cutting off their supply of nutrients. If algae grow out of control they can also block tubes and fittings. Though there are some natural water additives that can inhibit the growth of algae, namely grapefruit seed extract and hydrogen peroxide for more established plants, prevention is always the best medicine. Blocking as much light from the inner workings of your system is an effective means of algae control, as they can't live in darkness. In single-planter systems (like the small-scale set-up below), the planters can be covered with light-proof film, plastic, or aluminum foil, with holes poked out for the plants. Make sure that the growing media, tubing, and reservoir are either wrapped or in a cabinet, or placed inside of commercial anti-algae bags.

Four sets of instructions follow: 1 and 2 - the small and large scale set-ups, 3 - bucket and drum growing, and 4 - the growing wall, or vertical garden. The smaller set-up consists of individually flooding containers, can be put together in a couple of hours with a single trip to a hardware store, and are a low-commitment and small-space way to get started with a few herbs, tomato or strawberry plants. The larger system will utilize a large "bath" that plants can easily be put into and taken out of, and will be more expensive (though still under $100) and require more handiness, but if you're serious about growing food and have the space (for two plastic totes, which can be stacked on top of each other, so not super huge), I recommend you jump right into this one. Bucket and Drum growing are a little more industrial and do best in a greenhouse situation, or at least a large room that gets flooded on at least 2 sides with sunlight for several hours a day. Same thing with the Vertical Garden, though if you have the light (natural or artificial) it will turn a wall into a breathtaking cascade of greenery and nutriment. The important thing here is that the simple concept of flooding and draining roots with nutrient-rich water is the same, and if after reading through all the plans you want to hybridize them or create a system that's completely your own, more power to ya.

Small-Scale Set-Up

This system is designed to go in front of a window. If you don't have adequate light for fruiting plants (if that's what you're going with), your window space is already being used for grasses or micro-lettuces, or you'd just like to put the system elsewhere for esthetic reasons, check out the section on artificial light. It's very quick and easy to get up and running, and finding sources for the equipment is by far the most time-consuming part (but I've tried to help you out in "Resources").

What you'll need: (unless you have a friend who works at a hydro store, it's cheapest and easiest to get everything but the bottles online, but the stores that would carry the individual things are listed for your covenience)

Recycling center or neighbor's garbage:

3 or more 2 liter soda bottles with caps. The bottoms will be cut off, the bottles turned upside down, and the opening will hold the plant.

Pet Store:

Aquarium pump, 1 psi or the smallest/cheapest you can find

1 ft of ¼" air tubing

Hardware Store/Lumber Yard/Nursery:

2 ft of 3/8" vinyl or plastic irrigation tubing, add a foot for every extra soda bottle planter

A number of 3/8" barbed plastic "T" adapters, 1 for every bottle, minus the last one. Also called barbed hose fitting, and available in nylon.

1 - 3/8" barbed plastic elbow, see above

13 feet of 1x4 lumber – 1 @ 32", 4 @ 28", and 4 @ 3 ½"; the lumber yard can cut them for you if you don't have a saw, for 25-50 cents per cut, though if you ask nicely they may waive the fee

1 - Piece of plywood or melanine, 32" x 28". This is the front cover and is just for looks, so can be skipped or made as pretty as you like. I'll leave it up to you how you want to attach the cover; anything from just leaning it against the legs, to a loose nail that can be pushed in and out, to hinges that allow you to swing open your apparatus and wow your book club, will do fine. The sides can also be covered for noise reduction and looks – add more material as needed.

24 - 2" drywall screws

(Hydroponics store or internet):

Growing Medium (See chapter XX for more info about soilless growing mediums, but there's one extra thing to think about when choosing one for your project: density. The more air there is in your medium, the more water you'll need to fill it up, and the larger your reservoir tank will need to be. Pea Gravel is a good solution for hydro growing: cheap and packs tightly.)

Plants and nutrients

Tools:

A tube of silicon caulk

Utility knife

Measuring tape

Drill with a screw bit and 7/32, 3/8, and 1-1/4 inch bits. I cringe at the thought of you buying a drill for this project – you'd have to grow a lot of tomatoes before you came out ahead. Maybe you know someone who has one you can borrow or trade for sprouts.

Drilling and cutting:

Drill 3/8" holes in the center of all the bottle caps, and an additional 7/32" hole in one (for the reservoir). Make sure to leave room for the threads of the bottle when it's screwed on.

Cut the ends of the tubing at angles to make it easier to stick them through the holes.

Cut the bottoms off of all the 2 liter bottles but one (the reservoir). Poke multiple holes in the bottom and invert it inside the bottle to hold the growing medium. Depending on the size of the growing medium you're using, you may also want to use a plastic produce bag with many holes poked in it, and the opening rubber banded or paper clipped to the opening in the bottle. [Side Note – Sunlight Dishwashing Liquid comes in bottles that are smaller than

2 liters but have nipples underneath the pop-out dispenser tops that fit 3/8" tubing perfectly. If you'd prefer growing a larger number of smaller plants or can't find barbed connectors and have a source for these bottles, go for it.]

Drill 1 ¼" holes in the 32" piece of 1x4, 5 ½" inches from each end and 4" apart. This will give you 5 holes.

Quick and Easy Assembly

Apply silicon on all wet connections

Screw 1x4 pieces together to form the case as shown

Feed about a foot of the 3/8" tubing and an inch of the ¼" tubing through the top of the cap of the reservoir bottle, the one with two holes

Place elbow and "T" connectors through bottle caps and screw onto bottles.

Invert bottles through holes in cross-beam, the one with the elbow connector at one end

Connect the bottles together using 3/8" tubing with enough length so they won't pull on the connectors, but short enough so as not to form a "U" in between connections. The elbow connector is on one end, the "T" connectors are in the middle, and the reservoir is on the other end, standing on the ground.

Connect the reservoir and aquarium pump with the ¼" tubing

Getting It Going:

Rinse your growing medium until the run-off it clear, and put it in the planters with a plant. If you're using a potted plant, gently rinse off any soil with in a sink or with a hole. Put a layer of growing medium in the bottom of the planter, then hold the plant in place with one hand while gently sprinkling in the rest of the medium until the plant is secure.

Make some nutrient water, and while putting a kink in the 3/8" tube between the last planter and the reservoir (you may want to bend it and cinch it with a rubber band or have a friend hold it) fill the planters to just below the top of the growing medium. Then take out the kink so that the water drains into the res. This is the best way to make sure you have the right amount of water. If the reservoir fills up, there's too much water in the system and it could back up into the pump, which will ruin it. See if you can use a denser, or less, growing medium. About half to three-quarters full is a good level. Time how long it takes all the water to drain out.

Plug in the pump. The air fills up the reservoir and pushed the water up into the planters. Time how long it takes to do this, then unplug the pump and time how long it takes to drain. The two times added together are one cycle, probably around 2 minutes. Set the timer to 3-5 cycles per day, if you're using one. If any water or air leaks out, drain the system and use the silicon on the offending openings.

Large-Scale Hydro Set-up

The idea behind this system is the same as the last: nutrient-rich water washes over the roots of growing medium-suspended plants at pre-ordained intervals. The difference is that instead of having a few-inch-in-diameter planter for each plant, the large-scale set-up uses one large, shallow basin as a shared planter, with room for dozens or hundreds of plants. You'll notice that the list of supplies and steps to assemble is about the same size in both recipes.

What You'll Need:

2 Plastic Tubs...

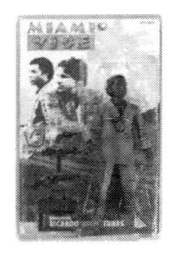

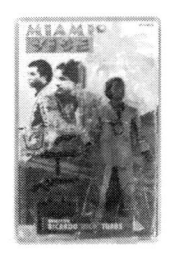

...just kidding

They should be at least 1 ½ ft by 2 ft, and if one has a lid, and the other is half as deep or more (at least 7 inches) and can sit on top of the deep one, so much the better. The deep lidded one will be the reservoir and the shallow one on top will be the growing tray. If you're going the stacked, small footprint route, make sure that the lid can handle a hundred pounds of weight, and that you can handle a hundred pounds when you have to move the growing tray to get to the reservoir, like when you change the water every two weeks. Otherwise, cinderblocks or a sturdy shelf or rack can hold the growing tray up higher than the res.

A Submersible Pump

This is the heart of the system. Get one that's rated at least 200 Gallons Per Hour (GPH). There are two other things that matter: "x-feet head", and "psi". The "head" tells us how far the pump can pump; if it's less than 4 feet, the length of our tubing, it might be the little engine that couldn't so play it safe and get the stronger model. If you want to expand in the future, you will be glad you did. Acceptable models start at $20-$30.

An Aquarium Air Pump and Air Stone, or Bubbler, with tubing.

This will oxygenate your nutrient water to prevent settling and stagnation, and are often available as a unit. This item isn't absolutely necessary, especially if you can create a splash when the upper tub drains into the lower.

2 Elbow Fittings, called *"Plastic Mushroom Head" or* , "90 degree through-wall fittings"

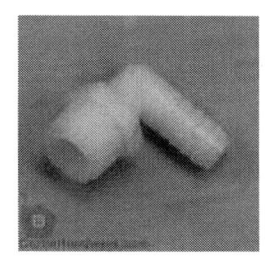

These are *"barbed"* so that tubing can be attached, are plastic, nylon, or brass, and they come with a nut on the other side so they can be secured to the wall of your tray. Try to find the same size barbs as your submersible pump so that the tubing will fit without an adapter, but if you can't it's an easy fix.

Tubing, 4 kinds:

1 - For your aquarium pump, if it didn't come with

2 – 5 feet, to go from your barbed fittings to your submersible pump. If they're not the same size, get an adapter or resizing tube that will allow 2 different-sized tubes to be connected together.

3 – 5 feet, twice the diameter of the above tube

4 - 6 inches of stiff plastic tubing with the end of the tube covered with a wide-mesh screening material (like window screen) and rubber-banded in place

A Timer, Growing Medium, Nutrients, and Plants

Tools: a drill with a 3/8" bit, and a tube of silicon caulk

Assembly

Drill 2 holes in the shallow growing tray, just wide enough to fit the barbed fittings through. They should both be in the center of one end of the tray; one as close to the bottom as possible (but make sure you leave enough room to screw the nut on the fitting) and the other 6 or 7 inches up. It's easier to drill through thin plastic if you hold a board or piece of wood against the other side of the wall.

Insert the fittings into these 2 holes so that the barbs are on the outside pointing down, apply silicon to both sides, and screw on the nuts.

Drill 3 holes in one end of the lid of the bigger container; 2 for tubing and one for power cords.

Insert the stiff plastic tube into the lower fitting from the inside. This will keep debris out of the reservoir, and will assist drainage (by the "capillary effect"; the surface tension created by liquids in thin tubes adds extra suction which even allows water to flow uphill, and this will keep liquid from pooling at the bottom of your growing tray. You've seen this cool phenomenon when soaking up water from a countertop with a paper towel; tiny pores in the fabric "wick" up many times their weight in liquid. This was the subject of Einstein's first paper.)

Connect the submersible pump to the upper fitting, running the tubing through one of the holes in the lid. Connect a piece of tubing from the bottom fitting and run it through another hole in the lid. Run the power cord of the submersible pump through the third hole in the lid, and put the pump in the reservoir tub. DO NOT PLUG IT IN YET.

Put everything you've constructed so far where it's going to live. Make sure that the place you choose can support a few hundred pounds. If you're not putting the growing tray on top of the reservoir, put it on a sturdy shelf or platform that's at least as high as the top of the reservoir.

Rinse your growing medium until the run-off it clear, and put it in the growing tray, about 6" deep.

Put a kink in the drainage hose, clamp or rubber band it, and fill up the growing tray until the water is about an inch below the surface of the growing medium. Record how much water it took to do this. Un-kink the hose and let it rain.

Because your growing medium was already wet, you know how much water is in the reservoir, and therefore how much nutrient solution to add to it. If you lost track, you can measure down from the rim, empty the water out, and fill it back up to the mark, taking note of how many gallons you've used. Add your nutrient solution. In the future, you may want to make your own solution, but with different nutritional needs at different stages, for different plants, and in different climates, I recommend you get the hang of hydro first. Here's a great resource when you're ready for it: www.motherearthnews.com is a great database for homemade nutrient solutions – search "hydroponic nutrients".

Plant your plants! If you're using starters that were formerly in soil, gently rinse it all away, then bury the roots in the growing medium. In hydroponics, plants can be put much closer together than in soil - you can plant them half the recommended distance apart.

Plug in the submersible pump. The pump sucks water in from the reservoir and pushes it into the grow tray. Time how long it takes to do this, then unplug the pump, and time how long it takes to drain. The two times added together are one cycle, probably around 20-30 minutes. Set the timer to 5-8 cycles per day. Watch your plants to see if they droop (not enough water) or turn yellow (too much water), and adjust accordingly.

If you're using the aquarium pump, it will sit outside of the system, so run its tube through one of the holes and plug it in.

With a powerful enough submersible pump and a "T" fitting in the filling tube, this system can easily expand to two growing trays and beyond.

The Growing Wall

Both the Growing Wall and the Barrel Garden, which follows, require more technical skill than the smaller hydro set-ups, though only about half as much as putting together a bookcase from IKEA. For the Growing Wall, each of the 3 main steps: 1) assembling the wooden frame and PVC planters, 2) assembling the lower pipes, 3) setting up the irrigation tubing and pump, are separated into their own section, each has its own materials list and assembly instructions. It's best to look through the entire plan before you get started, then buy all materials for all 3 steps at once.

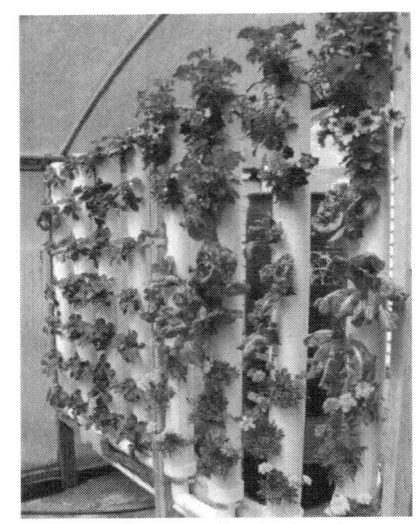

Step 1 - Frame and Planters

Step 1 Materials:

2-3" tape; masking, painters, duct, whatever.

Marker or grease pencil (a different color than the PVC)

A heat gun or powerful hair dryer

Saw, circular or hack (see Cutting the PVC, paragraph 2)

Nice but not necessary:

A spray bottle with water

PVC:

About a foot of 1.25" PVC (1.5" will also work)

4 – 57"' lengths of 4" thinwall (Schedule 20) PVC (buy 2 - 10' lengths, available in white or black; do you want your wall garden to be ninja or samurai?)

[Note – you need to be able to reach the top of the tube, and if you're a shorty and don't want to use a stepstool, plan ahead. The tubes will start at 2 feet from the ground, so measure how much higher than that you can reach and cut the PVC accordingly. Then read and understand these instructions so you'll know what other mods to make before you start.

Note 2 - If you don't own a saw or don't feel like cutting, you can buy 3 - 96" 2x4's and 2 - 10' lengths of PVC and ask them to cut them to the appropriate lengths for you. I'd keep a measuring tape with me and use it (you can borrow one from the store while you're in it) to make sure the cuts are accurate, or to inspire the cutter to make them so.]

Wood for the frame:

2 – 80" 2x4's

1 – 43" 2x4

1 – 40" 2x4

If you'd like to give the frame a coat of paint or other finish, now's the time.

Step Assembly:

Cutting the PVC

We'll be staggering the planting holes so we can fit more of them. Run a piece of tape that's 2 or 3 inches thick from one end of the tube to the other. Lay your measuring tape on the tape and make a mark at 2". Make a mark on the other side of the tape, 6" away from the first mark. Continue to mark every 6", alternating sides, until you have 9 marks. [One side of the tape: 2", 1'2", 2'2", 3'2", and 4'2". The other side of the tape: 8", 1'8", 2'8", and 3'8"]

Repeat on the other 3 PVC tubes, and remove the tape.

Next, we'll be cutting slots horizontally in the tube when it's standing up (crosswise), with the mark we just made in the center. Measure and mark or eyeball 2 ½" lines on the marks, and cut them with an electric circular saw or hack saw. The latter is much easier to control if you're not tool proficient, but will take a little longer. It's even more of a chore, but if you don't want to spend the $15 for a hack saw you can just buy a blade, make a handle by wrapping a rag around one end, and hold it while you saw. If you're using a circular saw, use a plywood blade turned backwards, so the teeth don't catch the surface. Then set the base plate to allow 2 ½", front-to-back, of the blade to stick out. Wear eye and face protection to keep smoke or shards out of you.

The end of the PVC pipe that has a slot 2" away from the edge is the top, and the end with the slot 8" away from the edge is the bottom.

Making the planting pockets

With your glue gun or hair dryer, heat one of the slots in an oval, about 3" wide and 5" high. Keep moving the heat so that the PVC doesn't brown or smoke (see PVC safety section on page XX). Keep heating until the PVC is soft and pliable. It will be hot so use something to poke it besides your finger.

By sticking your 1.25" or 1.5" piece of PVC into the slits, make pockets by pulling the bottom lip out and pushing the top lip in. Work the PVC into the pocket and firmly pull it towards you like a lever to position each lip properly. Make sure the pockets are hanging straight out from the surface of the PVC, not at a jaunty angle. Wait for it to cool down; spraying it with water will speed the cooling. Repeat on the other slots, making sure that they're oriented the right direction. If you mess up, the pocket can easily be re-heated and re-formed.

Keep the heat away from the very ends of the tubes so they don't deform. It's not easy to get them back in shape.

Step 2 - Assembling the lower pipes

Step 2 Materials:

PVC glue

4 - 4" to 2" PVC reducers with schedule 20 (thinwall) to schedule 40 (thickwall) adapters. (Some reducers have the adapters built-in, if you don't find those just buy 4" thin-to-thick adapters separately and glue them in the 4" opening of the reducer.)

2" PVC:

4 – 2" PVC at 2" long

2 – 2" PVC at 3" long

2 – 2" PVC at 10" long

3 – 2" PVC "T" fittings

1 square foot of plastic "cut your own" air conditioner filter

2' Plumbers strap

Step 2 Assembly:

Attach 2 of reducers to the "T" fittings. Connect the 2" side of the reducers to the "T" fitting by sliding the 2" long piece of 2" PVC into both openings. Make sure that the "T" and reducer touch, if not, shorten the 2" piece until they do. When everything fits together well, take them apart, glue all touching surfaces, and put them together permanently.

Repeat with the other 2 reducers and the "L" fittings. Glue the 10" lengths of 2" PVC into the openings of the "L" fittings.

Cut 4" round circles out of the air conditioner filter material by laying the 4" bell of the reducer n top of it and cutting around it with a utility knife. The round filter pieces goes inside of the 4" bell of the reducers. This will keep the growing medium in the planting tube and out of the water reservoir.

Lay the "T"s and "L"s down flat on a surface. The "T"s go in the middle and the "L"s go on the ends, with the openings towards the middle. There needs to be 11" in between the fittings, center-to-center, so insert the end of the 10" long 2" PVC from the "L" into the "T" fitting, marking it at the appropriate distance and cutting if necessary. Glue them together and quickly align the reducers so they're pointing the same direction. One way to do this is to put the 4" bells down on a flat surface and make sure both the top edges of the bells touch all the way around. You now have one "TL" assembly. Make another "TL" assembly with the other "T" and "L" fittings.

Glue the 3" pieces of 2" PVC into the other end of the "T"s, so you can attach the last "T" fitting in between them, this time pointing the exact opposite direction. This will be the drain. You'll have to do this by eye. Make sure that, as before, the middle "T"/reducer assemblies are exactly 11" apart, center-to-center, cutting the 2" PVC if necessary.

Attach the finished reducer assembly to the frame

Lay the frame down with the horizontal 2x4's on the ground. Position the finished reducer assembly against the lower 2x4, with the 4" bells up and the bottom edges of the bells resting on the top of the 2x4". Wrap a length of plumbers strap around the reducers so that the ends can be screwed into the 2x4, holding the assembly in place. The strap can be cut to the proper length with shears or bent backwards and forward several times until it snaps off. Attach the strap to the 2x4 and put 2 screws in each end, as these straps will be holding the weight of the planters, growing medium, and plants, then put a screw as close in to the corner as possible to tighten it down.

Insert the 4" planting tubes into the reducers, making sure that the front (where the tape was) is pointing straight out. When you like the fit, glue it.

The top of the planting tubes should be even with the top of the wood frame. Make sure that the tubes are 11" apart all the way up. Put a screw through the inside of the tube into the top horizontal 2x4.

Step 3 - Setting up the irrigation tubing and pump

Step 3 Materials:

15' of ½" black irrigation tubing

½" electrical conduit brackets (black plastic cuffs with nails sticking out that we'll use to attach the irrigation tubing to the wood frame.)

1/8" tubing poker (in the irrigation section of the hardware store)

Growing medium. Can be scavenged roadside gravel, coarse sand if you're by a beach, or pumice (spongy lava rock) if you live near a volcano, but perlite is recommended because it's very light and cheap. Vermiculite, pea gravel, and clay pebbles are also good options. You'll need 90 quarts of medium, which, just to give you an idea, is 30 pounds of perlite ($30-$40).

Submersible Pump with at least a 7' lift, which will be 150-600 gallons per hour of flow.

You'll also probably need an adapter so your pump can connect to the 1/8" tubing, as they usually as designed to fit a garden hose.

Choosing a pump - how high it can pump the water (the head) is much more important than the volume of water it can pump (the flow). Sometimes, the head isn't listed, but you should be safe with at least a 200 GPM pump. These start at around $35 (check ebay), but pumps with better warranties and similar specs can go for over $300. If your cheaper pump croaks, you'll have to water by hand until your new one comes. Worth the savings I think.

Drill and a 3/16" bit

Breathing mask

Step 3 Assembly:

Turn the frame and PVC assembly around so that the back of the horizontal 2x4s and the smooth side of the PVC is facing you. Leaving a few inches of the ½" irrigation tubing sticking out to the left, attach it along the underside of the top horizontal 2x4 with the ½" electrical conduit brackets every foot or so. When you get to the right side, you won't be able to put a 90 degree angle in the irrigation tubing without kinking it, so just go as far as you can and then start attaching it to the back of the vertical 2x4 on the right.

The tubing will go behind the upside-down "T" fitting in the middle of the "LTTTL" assembly and into the bucket, so make sure when you attach it that there's room for both corners, without kinking.

To cap off the open end of the tubing at the upper left, kink it at the edge of the wood and fold it back on itself. Use 2 nylon zip-ties to attach it to THE PTHER TUBE so that no water can spray out of that end. Trim the ends of the zip-ties and turn the thing around to face you.

Using your 1/8" tubing poker, poke 2 holes in the ½" irrigation tubing in between the planting tubes and one on each side of the far right and left tubes. The holes can be evenly spaced for esthetic reasons. Cut 8 pieces of 1/8" irrigation tubing about a foot long. Cut the ends at 45 degrees so that they won't seal against the back of the larger tube and block the water flow; it also makes them easier to insert. Put them into the holes you poked.

Drill 3/16" holes in both sides of all the planting tubes. Position the drill bit about 1 or 1 ½" from the top and start to slowly drill. When the bit catches, move the drill so that you're drilling down at about 45 degrees. Insert the free ends of the 1/8" tubing into these holes, so that each planting tube has 2 water inlets, just in case one gets clogged.

[During Use: Check the pipes every so often by pulling them out of the PVC and confirming that they're squirting water out at the normal volume. If they're not, pull the other end out, turn it around, and reattach it, so that reversing the direction of flow will blow out the clog.]

Fill the planting tubes with your growing medium. It's a little dusty, depending on your medium, and messy, depending on your pouring skills. It's best to do this as close as possible to where your wall is going to live, but if you have to fill it outside and have a friend help you carry it in, take a picture of yourselves negotiating the elevator and send me a copy.

[On choosing a spot: if the wall is going to be inside next to a real wall, it can be screwed though the top 2x4 to hold it up. It can also be held upright in this way on the outside of a building, or against an eave or tree (though maybe you can use a rope instead of a screw). If it is to be free-standing, attach 3 foot 2x4s to the legs as a base, with angled 2x4s or upside-down shelf brackets, or angle irons to brace it. Make sure to secure the wall somehow if it could be hit by a gust of wind. If your bucket is going to be in the sun, be careful that it doesn't heat up too much. Putting something reflective around it will help keep it cool, but putting up a shade screen is even better, and of course, you'll want to cover it to keep dirt and bugs out.]

The easiest way to fill the tubes is to prop the Growing Wall at an angle, fill a bucket with the medium, and pour it into the tubes. Make sure you're wearing a breathing mask. When you've filled the tubes as much as you can at an angle, straighten the wall and top them off.

Put your wall in its final destination. Fill the 5 gallon bucket with nutrient water and put it underneath the drain "T". The drain can be run elsewhere if your growing wall is a work of art, and you don't want the bucket in view. Use a reducer and 2" PVC to drain the water wherever you want, making sure that there's enough downward grade in the pipe for the water to drain. Put your bucket in a box on the side of the wall, around a corner, or even through the wall behind it into a closet, which will minimize the sound as well.

Connect your pump to the 1/8" tubing, with a clamp if necessary, but don't plug it in yet. Gently place it onto the bottom of the bucket, plug it in, and say a little prayer. If you've done everything correctly, you will hear a gurgling, feel a slight vibration in the wall, and in 15 minutes will find dampness in the topmost pockets. As things go on, watch the level of your bucket; depending on the growing medium you've chosen, you'll have to add more nutrient water to the bucket to keep the pump submerged. In an hour and a half, you should be able to find wetness in all the pockets, and the water level in the bucket will stay steady as the all the medium has become fully saturated.

The Growing Wall is ready to be planted. (Or maybe, now that you're a pro, you'd like to build a few more walls first.)

Planting the Wall

With a blunt object, like the handle of a paintbrush or screwdriver, make a hole in one of the pockets by pushing the medium out of the way in all directions. Take the plant's roots (all the dirt rinsed off if you're using plants started in soil) and gently put it into the hole, letting its roots spread out as much as possible. Fill in any gaps with more growing medium (you can steal it from the top of the tube) and you're all set. Be careful when planting in the bottom pockets that you don't disturb the filter.

Barrel and Drum Gardening

Materials:

A Barrel

Medium Marker

Straight Edge as tall as your barrel

Measuring tape

A way to cut out slits in the barrel, whether a circular saw, utility knife, router, or something else, but a circular saw with the plate adjusted for a 4" cut is the fastest

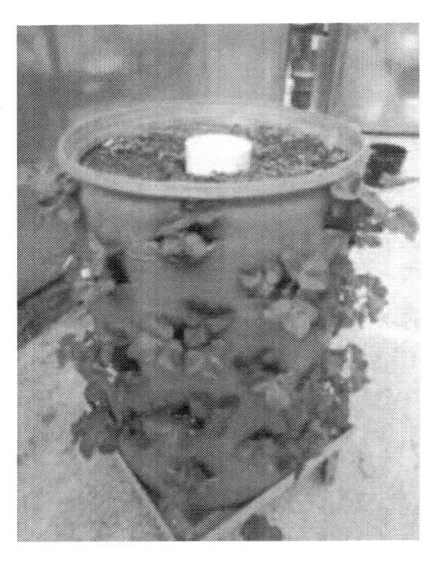

Choosing your barrel

Size Options:

Any size barrel can be used, and the biggest that will fit your space is recommended. If the barrel might need to be moved, it can be put on a garbage can roller. A 55 gallon barrel has room for 80 plants plus a 4 foot square area on top, a 5 gallon 25 plants, a little less than 1 square foot. 300 gallon barrels are also available.

If you decide to go with a used barrel, keep in mind what it was used for. No pesticides, paint, or other chemicals. Food use is best.

Remove or cut off top and clean off the edges with a knife. Cut the lid off down from the top as opposed to from the side, to keep the strong ring that runs along the top of the barrel just below the upper edge.

We'll be making growing cells 4" apart all over the barrel, which is too close together for most plants. When we discuss planting in the barrel, we'll be skipping cells vertically to allow for more room for roots, either every other cell for strawberries, lettuces, peppers, etc, or every third cell for larger plants like squash, larger tomato varieties, and cucumbers. 4" apart is fine for herbs and non-fruiting plants like that. We're making planting cells in this way to allow for the most flexibility in choosing and planting plants, but if you know for sure that you're only going to be using your barrel garden for larger plants, save time by making the rows 12" apart.

Measure around the barrel and top to bottom to find out how much surface area you have to determine how many rows, columns, and total planting cells you're going to have. For example, a 55 gallon drum is 36" high and 75" in circumference. If you use cells 4" apart, you'll have room for 7 cells in a vertical column and 18 in a horizontal row, 84 total. Now you know how far from the top and bottom to make your cuts, at least 4", and in this example, exactly 4". Make sure there's an even number of marks in a horizontal row.

Wrap a measuring tape around the top of the barrel and mark every 4" with a dot. Using a vertical seam in the barrel, a straight edge, or a level, mark the bottom row of cells even with the top. Then, using your straightedge top-to-bottom or a pre-marked piece of string pulled tight between the top and bottom rows, mark the barrel every 4". Go around the barrel this way until you run out of room, and you will have a hive of intercrossing diagonals If it's not perfect, don't worry about it, because as long as there's maximum room for plants, the rest it just aesthetics.

Now, connect the dots. Draw a line between two dots in a horizontal row, then skip, then connect the next two, going all the way around like this. Because there's an even number in each row, we won't be left with a long space or a long line. Then do the next row down, but STAGGER the lines from the top so they don't line up vertically, like rows of bricks. This will give your plants' roots extra room. Keep connecting dots this way to finish this row, then continue down the barrel, staggering every row. If you're confident in your abilities, you don't need to connect the dots with marker, you can just cut away. But one daydream and you may end up with uneven rows. If you're super sneaky, you can make half as many marks in each row and center the saw blade when cutting.

Cut the slits. If you're using a circular saw, adjust the plate so that only 4" of blade is exposed, front-to-back. This way, when you put the front of the saw against the barrel's surface and lower the back down to cut the slit, you won't have to move the saw at all except for this downward motion. Heat and open the slits in the same way as in the growing wall instructions above, focusing more heat on the bottom lip than the top. It will take about 45 seconds to a minute to heat it, and the same to stretch and cool it. If you have 84 slits you're looking at an hour and half to two hours, so consider putting on a movie or getting another heat gun and a friend to help. It will speed things up as well if you make wedges out of 2x4s cut in half longways and at an angle to stick though the heated slits, to hold them in place as they cool.

Nearly any plant can be grown with an aeroponic growing system. Aeroponic plants grow faster, yield more, and are healthier than soil-grown plants. Aeroponics also requires little space, making it ideal for growing plants indoors. No growing medium is used with an aeroponic growing system. Instead, the roots of aeroponic plants are suspended in a darkened chamber, which is periodically sprayed with a nutrient-rich solution. One of the biggest drawbacks is affordability, with many commercial aeroponic growing systems being quite costly. That's why many people choose to make their own personal aeroponic growing systems.

DIY Aeroponics

There are actually many ways to create a personal aeroponic system at home. They are easy to construct and are by far less expensive. A popular DIY aeroponics system makes use of large, storage bins and PVC pipes. Keep in mind that measurements and sizes vary depending on your own personal aeroponic needs. In other words, you may need more or less, as this project is meant to give you an idea. You can create an aeroponic growing system using whatever materials you like and whatever size you want.

The following is instructions for a simple aero set-up, using a plastic tote container. The system is so simple that it can be easily modified to work with another container. An aeroponic hybrid of the Growing Wall, using vertical or horizontal PVC, is a simple modification.

The Aero-Tote

Materials:

A Heavy Duty Plastic Tote Container with Reinforced Lid. Make sure the lid has raised edges so any water overspray won't run off.

A Fountain Pump, 200 GPH (see pg 141 for more info on pumps). [A smaller cheaper pump might work as well, but the backpressure may become an issue]

4' - 1/2" Poly Tubing that's the same size as your pump's fittings, or adapters

3 - T-type Poly Connectors

6 to 12 - 360-degree misting or fogging Spray Nozzles with 1/4" fitting

4 - 8 1/4" poly tube extenders.

Hose Fitting to attach pump to 1/2" tube.

12" - Clear Vinyl Tube (this will be the water level indicator)

Angle connector, Misc connectors and Rubber Washers for Water Level Indicator.

30 to 40 2" Plastic Net Cups

30 to 40 - 2" Neoprene collars for net cups. Only about 35 cents each, but these can also be homemade.

Growing Medium, Plants, Organic Fertilizer (bat guano mixed with kelp or seawater is good)

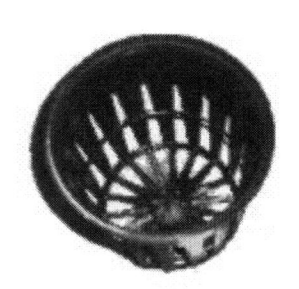

Optional:

EPDM Weather Stripping (to help seal the lid to the base, a good idea if the unit will be kept somewhere that can't get a little wet.)

Plastic Spring Clamps (Optional)

If your unit will drop below 60 degrees, add a small aquarium heater to the reservoir.

Tools Needed:

Drill with a 2" Hole Saw, Wire Brush Bit, and an (approx.) 5/8" bit

Sharpie for marking.

2 channel lock pliers to tighten fittings

Serrated knife or box cutter

Zip Ties

Assembly

Step 1 - Prepare the Plastic Lid:

Using the 2" hole saw and drill, cut as many holes as you can without cutting through the structural ribbing. You'll be able to fit more holes (and therefore plants) if you mark all of your holes first to make sure they are evenly spaced. [Make sure to keep the left-over plastic "doughnuts" - you can use these instead of the neoprene collars by cutting a slit from the center hole to the edge.]

Our final pattern looks like this. We end up with 40 holes this way.

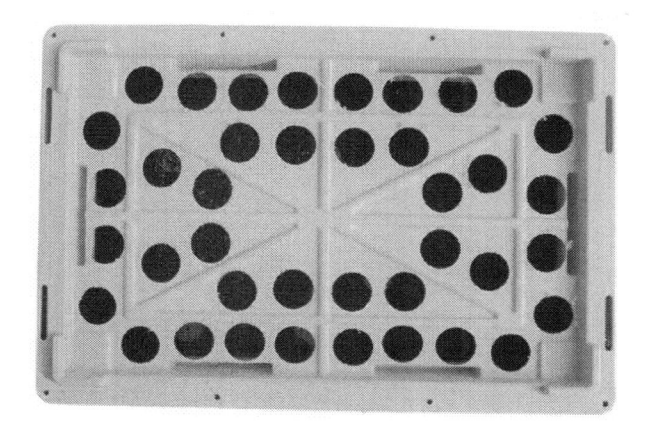

Use the wire brush to clean up the holes and remove the burrs. Don't use it too long in one spot or you'll melt the plastic.

Step 2 - Prepare the Water Level Indicator

The Water Level Indicator lets us know how much water is in the reservoir without having to remove the lid to check.

Cut a small hole near the bottom of the reservoir. The size will depend on the thread size of the connector pieces you have, ours was 5/8".

Attach the fittings with a rubber washer on the inside.

Attach the clear vinyl tube and secure it by drilling 2 small holes in the handle of the reservoir and securing it with a zip tie.

Step 3 - Tubing, Pump and Nozzle Assembly

The exact sizes for your tubing will depend on the size of your reservoir. Measure the inside of your container length times width, subtract 4" from both the length and width of your containing, and multiply the two numbers together.

Use the Hose Connector and T fittings to create an "8" that is 4" less than the both the length and width of your container. The fitting are compression fittings, so no glue is required. Use a downward-facing T-fitting in the middle of the center tube to attach the pump, with enough vertical tubing that the "8" sits several inches above the water line. The pump will be completely submerged with several inches of water above it.

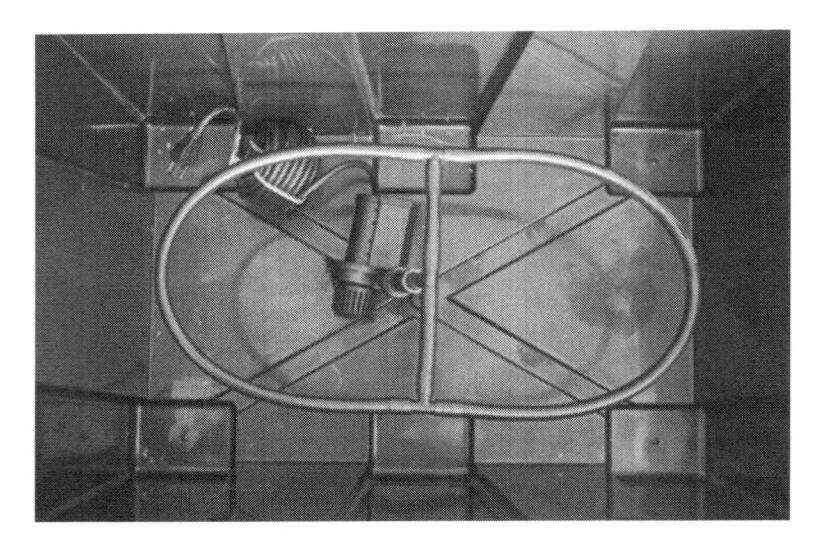

Attach the Spray Nozzles evenly around the "8". Insert the heads into the 1/2" Poly-tube by punching a small hole then threading on the heads. Direct the heads so that the spray will cover the entire area.

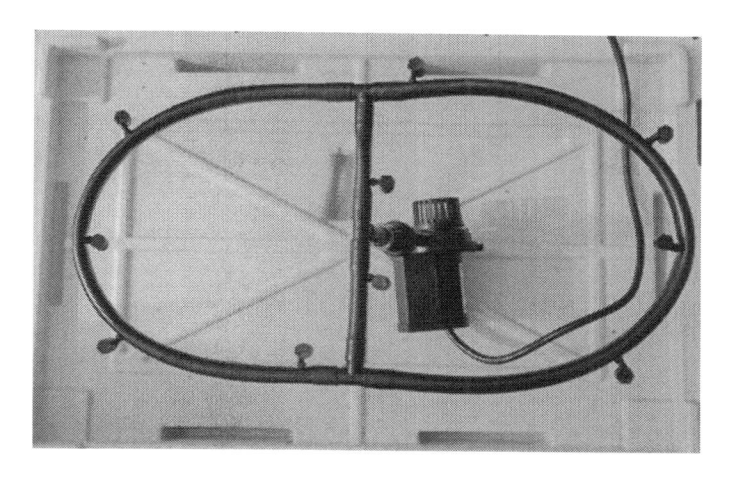

If your pump is unstable and wants to tip over, attach it to a plastic pot base by drilling two small holes and using zip ties to secure it.

Step 4 - Testing the system:

Clean the reservoir well. Any bits of plastic or dirt may clog the pump or spray heads. Fill the Tank with water, enough to cover the pump by a few inches.

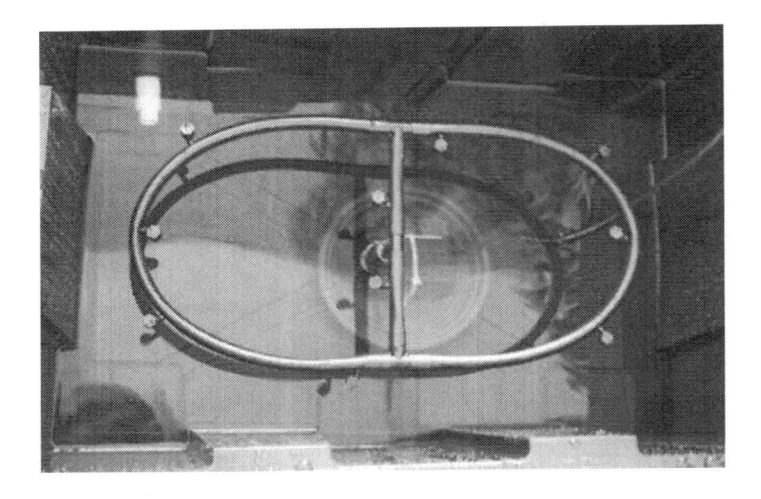

Plug the pump in and look for any areas that don't receive spray.

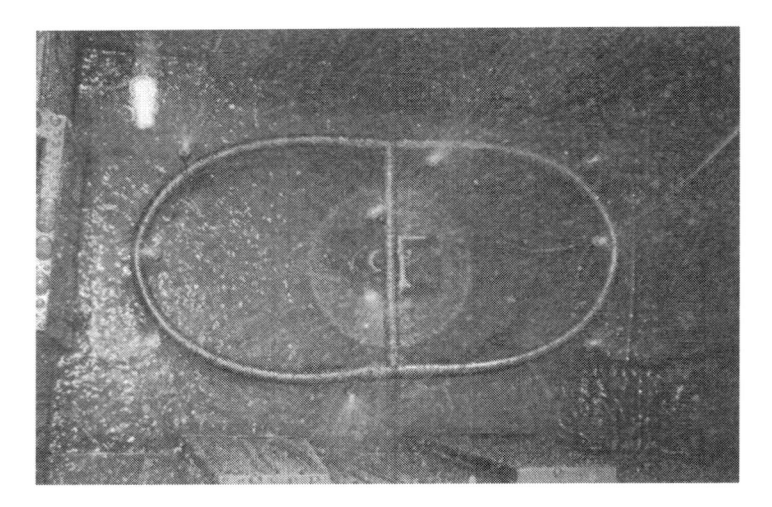

Step 5 - Assembly

Weather Strip the containers edge, if desired. Clean the lid, and run the weather stripping around the rim of the container. This step will prevent overspray from dripping down the sides of the unit.

Cut a hole in the side of the res to allow for a place to run the power cord, slotting the lid if necessary.

Secure the lid down with the spring clamps.

Insert your Net Pots and Neoprene Collars or Plastic Donuts. Pull out that Sharpie and mark your water level on the clear tube.

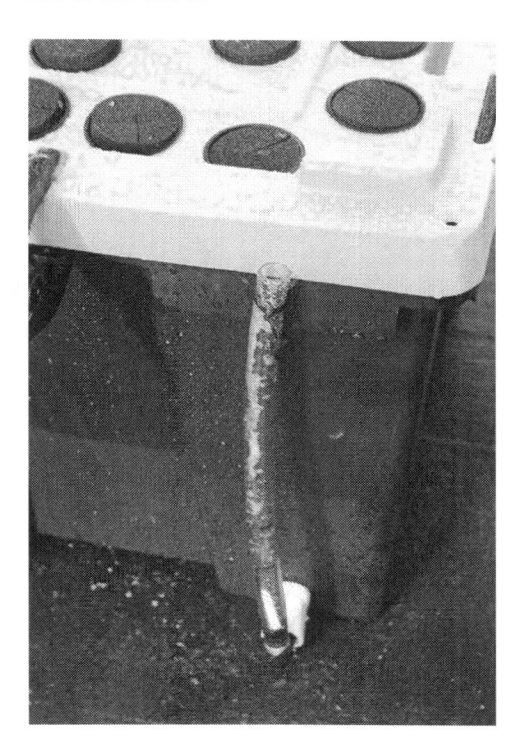

Step 6 - Operation

Test the unit one more time with the Net Cups in place, and see if they're getting wet. If you have a few dead spots, added a few more spray heads, to get full coverage. Spinner-type heads may give the most thorough watering.

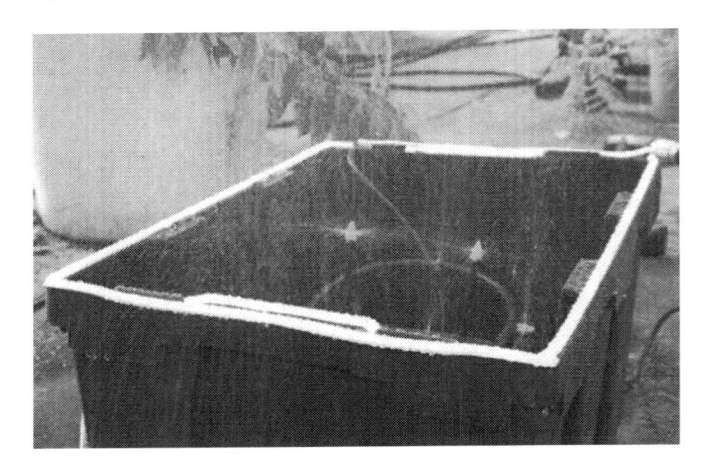

Fill the net cups with growing medium and add your plants. If they are coming from dirt, rinse the roots completely. Add fertilizer to the water. The unit will need to be cleaned with hydrogen peroxide (see pg XX) or diluted bleach after each cycle to prevent algae, fungus, and bacteria.

Composting and Worm-iculture

A forest is the ultimate self-sustaining garden. I grew up in the rural Midwest, and was lucky enough to have a backyard bordered by many acres of mucky woods. I spent a lot of my childhood back there amongst the living mud, crumbling branches, and moldering leaves, and often thought about the difference between the dirt there and in our yard-locked garden, just a hundred feet away. Have you ever noticed the dark, rich, and loamy soil in the woods? And how cracked, dry, and blonde a recently abandoned garden will become? No one needs to water or fertilize the woods.

Decay is La Différence. A forest floor is covered in decomposing matter: leaves, the spongy trunks of fallen trees, the fur, feathers, and bodies of dead animals and bugs. Microorganisms and worms in the ground recycle this and any other formerly-living matter into stable soil capable of feeding the next generation of growth. The tree canopy shields the forest floor from harsh sunlight, sprinkling it with a soft green glow. Exactly the right amount of moisture is retained for the native flora. If I would have taken a cactus and tried to plant it out there, it would have taken in as much water as possible, planning to store it for the next dry spell which would never come, and it would burst. A jade houseplant would have rotted with too much water. Likewise, plant a maple tree in a mountain pine forest, where the trees have developed tiny needles to gather sunlight and retain moisture, and it will wither and die while the plants around it will continue to thrive in their own way.

A forest can even purge itself of toxins and harmful chemicals. The composting process can neutralize volatile organic compounds (VOCs), bind heavy metals and render them inert, and even eliminate wood preservatives, pesticides, hydrocarbons, and explosives. I was once walking in the woods in Maryland and found a section along an ancient trail that was littered with old glass jars from before my time. This was early spring, the trees were slowly waking up from their winter sleep and the ground was still thawing and barren. But inside of every one of the jars the green leaves of little plants were unfolding alongside bright emerald mosses and delicate mushroom caps. I imagined that these unlikely terrariums found springtime before the rest of the forest every year, protected from the cold winds and enjoying sun-warmed, moist air. These plants must have grown too large for their containers and found their way out of the opening while the rest of the forest was just beginning to BLOOM, adding moisture to the forest climate and extending early invitations to animals and birds that would add their valuable influence to pollination and fertilization. These jars had in fact extended the growing season of this arboreal garden by a few weeks, and allowed for that many more fruits, seeds and grams of compost to be produced. The forest had found a way to deal with the most toxic influence of all, that of inconsiderate humans, in a way that added to its communal prosperity and evolutionary advantage.

In the same way, permaculture, the approach to designing agricultural systems that mimic nature, is sometimes whimsically called "lazy agriculture" by its practitioners. This isn't a jab at modern hippiedom but an appreciative awareness that if Nature is given a toehold, it will seize command. Once we establish a garden with even the slightest opportunity for sustainability, natural law will take over and very little effort is required by us to keep it "growing".

There are several different ways to put nature to work for you in making luscious new soil for your food-producing plants, and which you choose will depend mainly on your living arrangements. If you have yard space (and city ordinances allow it) then a traditional, low-maintenance compost heap is your best bet. A store-bought or homemade compost tumbler can go on a patio, balcony, or rooftop, and its sleek design and tight-fitting lid will keep its purpose and smell out of the minds and noses of neighbors, landlords, and pests. If you only have indoor space to work with, you can use what might be the most effective composting method of all: vermiculture, or worm composting. These guys will not only reduce the amount of food waste that goes into the garbage, they will also make a most delicious (to your plants, that is) fermented compost tea.

Even if you're more of a sprouter and fermenter and have little need for good dirt, keeping your kitchen scraps out of landfills and spreading your homemade soil in a local park or community garden is a very good deed. In a landfill, your kitchen wastes (which accounts for an average of a quarter of what people throw into the garbage, according to the EPA) decompose anaerobically (without oxygen), making methane, a greenhouse gas that's 72% more destructive than carbon dioxide, the gas that comes from burning coal and petroleum products. In a compost pile, the food and yard waste break down aerobically, producing a fraction of the methane. Since the 1700's methane in the Earth's atmosphere has gone up 150 times, while CO2 has increased "only" about 35 times (we know this from testing air bubbles in glaciers – very cool). Landfills are by far the largest source of atmospheric methane, with developed countries accounting for most of the production. Also, methane will be produced for years after a landfill is closed, as anaerobic decomposition of living matter is a much slower process than what happens in nature.

First, let's discuss how composting works. Layered compost piles mimic what happens on the forest floor, creating the ideal conditions for quick, natural breakdown. The process requires 4 ingredients: living matter, soil organisms, water, and air. During decomposition, bacteria, nematodes, and worms in the soil break down living matter into its simplest parts. This produces <u>fiber</u>-rich, carbon-containing **humus** with inorganic nutrients that plants can use.

Living matter is the main ingredient in the home compost heap, and it comes in two kinds:

1) "Green" - food scraps, lawn clippings, and fresh manure from vegetarian livestock, if you have access to it. Pet manure is fine if you make their food yourself or know exactly what goes in it. Seaweed, tea bags, and coffee grounds are great sources of supplemental nutrition to your pile, and attract a host of beneficial organisms. Meat, dairy, and oil however, are difficult to digest for a passive or new compost pile, and can create unpleasant odors. They're best added to a well-established, hot and oft-turned heap. Putting them through a blender or food-processor first will speed their decomposition, though some sources say that to avoid vermin in outdoor set-ups, meat and dairy should be skipped altogether. If any part of you is motivated to compost because of environmental factors, however, you may want to look into the negative global impact of raising animals for meat and forgo your bratwursts altogether. Crushed egg shells, however, are great additions in new compost piles.

2) "Brown" – dead leaves, newspaper, cardboard, pine needles, junk mail, dry straw and hay, and paper grocery bags. Greens have plenty of nitrogen while brown has more carbon, two essential nutrients for a thriving compost heap. The best ratio is 2 parts brown to 1 part green; a pile of dead leaves can take years to decompose without the heat of nitrogen, and a pile of kitchen scraps (or a jack-o-latern in November) without the drying carbon of brown matter will quickly turn into wet goo. A varied diet results in varied sources of plant matter to your compost, which will result in varied nutrients in your finished soil and food.

The following shouldn't go into your compost pile:

- **Diseased garden plants** - They can infect the compost pile and influence the finished product.
- **Invasive weeds** - Spores and seeds of invasive weeds (buttercups, morning glory, quack grass) can survive the decomposition process and spread to your plants when you use the finished compost.
- **Charcoal ashes** - toxic to the soil microorganisms.
- **Pesticide-treated plant material isn't great** – though it's an unreasonable requirement that food waste that goes into your compost heap be 100% organic, pesticides are harmful to the compost organisms and some types may survive in the finished compost. This especially applies to the particularly virulent ones that have been outlawed in America, and so are sold to developing countries and used on the fruit and produce that's then shipped back to us. Assuming the chapter on commercial farming did its job and you don't use conventionally-grown produce, if your less informed or more frugal neighbors donate their locally-grown kitchen scraps to your compost pile, then at least they stay out of landfills.

Soil microorganisms need water to live and oxygen to function. At the outset, dry brown matter should be thoroughly wetted, like a wrung-out sponge; afterwards the pile will generally take water out of the green matter and maintain its own moisture level that way. An exposed compost heap has easy access to air; prettier composting breathes well because of a good bin structure.

In an "open air" compost bin, made of wood pallets, chicken wire, or anything whose sole purpose is to keep out pests, respiration goes both ways and there will be an unpleasant smell. These structures are best in the corner of a yard, which obviously requires permission if you're in an apartment, condo, or rented house. Wood pallets are often available for free at any store that sells a lot of something:

Home Depot, Sam's Club, Target, Wal-mart, etc. Just go around back of the store and ask for some; they might tell you to come back at a certain time, after a delivery, but the big stores get several deliveries a day, so you'll probably get lucky. You'll need a minimum of 4, for a 4-sided bin, but if you have the space, you can add another 3-walled bin for every stage of the process: one for fresh material, one for partially composted matter, and the last for finished compost (10 pallets in all). Just dig a shallow square hole as wide as your structure, line 3 pallets up as walls and either screw them together or use bailing wire on the corners. Then use latch bolts on the fourth pallet to make a removable door, or just use more wire to make hinges and a twisted lock. If you're in a dry climate, you can speed up the compost process by stapling plastic sheeting around the inside of the bin with a separate sheet for the door, to keep in moisture.

This technique is known as passive composting, where the ingredients are piled up and nature is allowed to take its course. After the initial set-up the only effort required is removing the finished compost from the bottom and adding more food scraps on top, though the entire pile can be "harvested" at once if left to cook long enough. "Active composting" requires a little bit of daily effort, but is much faster and allows for an enclosed structure that mitigates smells. Whether it's tediously turning with a pitchfork or simply turning crank on a sleek tube depends on the bin.

A simple active outdoor composter can be made from an old plastic or metal trash can with a tight-fitting lid. Drill holes every few inches around the sides and bottom or punch them in with a hammer and nail to allow for ventilation. Then put the can on top of cinderblocks or paving stones to allow draining, especially important if you're using a rustable metal container. Layer in your 2 parts brown matter to 1 part green, making sure that the moisture level is like a wrung-out sponge. Put the can on its side and roll it back and forth for 30 seconds or so, until all its corporeal contents are thoroughly mixed, and put it up on the blocks. Repeat this every few days to a week, adding fresh material as desired.

It will take about 4-6 weeks for the compost to be finished, so choose the size of your can accordingly: 20-40 gallons is about right for a family.

If you don't have the yard space for Donkey Kong and need to keep your barrel in one spot while mixing, you can buy a compost tumbler for a few hundred bucks, or you can make your own in a couple of hours for less than $50.

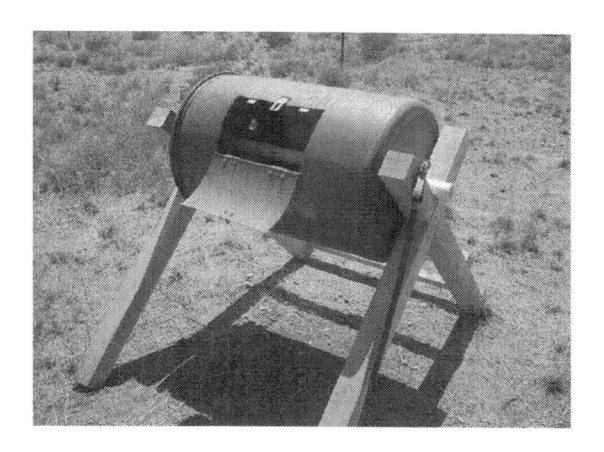

DIY Tumbling Composter

Get:

A plastic drum of 20-55 gallons (metal will work to, if you have to skills and tools to cut and drill it). All measurements in this recipe will deal with a 55 gallon drum, so alter the sizes to fit your barrel.

A 4' PVC pipe (a foot longer than your barrel), 1 ½ - 2 inches wide

5 pieces of metal rebar, 20" long

5 - 36" 2x4's (15' total board feet)

2" Drywall screws

A non-toxic epoxy that will bond pvc and metal

Tools: a utility knife, a drill with a ¼" bit, a bit the same diameter as the rebar, and a hole saw the same diameter as the PVC

Do:

Using the drywall screws, build 2 X's out of 4 the 2x4's, crossing them at right angles, and connect them halfway down one leg with the last piece of wood so they make a stand for the barrel on its side. If the tumbler is going to sit on a hard surface, cut the bottom ends of the X's so they're flat against the ground.

If your drum held anything potentially harmful to your compost, like cooking oil, wash it thoroughly. Don't use a barrel that held anything toxic like paint or petroleum.

Drill small holes all over the barrel, every few inches or so. (If you go with the "X" aesthetic theme mentioned below, you may want to drill cris-crossing bands of holes to form thick "X"s – purely cosmetic.)

Drill holes in the exact center of the lid and base of the barrel the same size as the PVC

Drill holes in the PVC just a bit smaller than the rebar, so that the metal rods sit snugly in place, even before they're glued. Drill a hole an inch from each end and 3 more holes evenly spaced that will be inside the barrel.

With the barrel on its side, cut a 3-sided flap in the side of the barrel about a foot and a half long (with the barrel on its side) and a foot tall. This will be the door. Attach a handle of some sort so it can be easily opened from the outside: an extra block of wood screwed on from the inside or glued, an old cabinet handle, whatever. You can also cut out all four sides and re-attach the bottom with hinges. If the plastic is so thin that the door pulls inside of the barrel, make the handle overhang the top edge of the flap so that it catches on the barrel and acts as a stop. Or get fancy and attach a "hasp" to the flap. This is a $1-2 piece of hardware with a loop on one side, and a flat piece of metal with a hole in it that goes over the loop on the other, often found on utility shed doors.

Insert the PVC in the hole in one of the round sides of the barrel. Insert all of the rebar through the holes in the PVC, inside of the barrel, except for the one an inch from the end. Epoxy the dead center of the rebar, and center the PVC so that the rebar sticks out evenly on each side. Put the other end of the PVC through the hole in the other side of the barrel, and epoxy the last pieces of rebar in the holes in the ends, outside of the barrel. These will be your cranks, turning your nouveau-pitchforks with ease. You only need to turn one crank at a time, the other one just keeping the end of the PVC outside the barrel. If you have a lot of compost mass, however, it helps to have two people turning, and this is a great way to involve a kid.

Lastly, instead of having a single rod as a crank, 2 rebars in the shape of an "X" on either side looks pretty cool and industrial, like a pirate ship's steering wheel or the hatch in "LOST", matches the "X"s in the wooden stands, and is slightly easier to turn. Totally up to you. Also, if you're not comfortable having a crank made out of potentially sharp, metally metal, you can make one out of PVC with 2 elbow fittings and 2 pieces of tubing, one at 12" and one at 6", standing with your side to the tumbler and grasping the short tube with two hands, turning it like an oar in a Viking longship. Cover the terminal end if you like with a PVC pipe cap or skip the short PVC and instead use a broken rake handle for the full Norse experience.

Your tumbling composter is ready to be filled with brown and green matter, wetted, and tumbled every few days.

If your tumbling will be conducted on a balcony or in a shared space and the earthy perfume is a concern, the device can be vented. Get a few feet of galvanized metal ducting from a hardware store, cut a hole to fit in the top of one or both sides of the barrel, and screw it on with a square plate fitment. Then (and this is the tricky part) buy some replacement filters for a home air purifier that have activated carbon. The expensive purifier appliance just pushes air through what really does the work, which is the inexpensive activated carbon. Stuff some of these sheets into the duct tubing, and you've made an apparatus for a few bucks that will drastically reduce the composting smell. Coffee grounds in the compost will also help.

Worm-i-culture

The most efficient composting, especially for apartment dwellers, is accomplished by worms in a cooperative procedure called "vermiculture". They will do all the tumbling and aerating, removing the need to turn compost by hand, and they will work year-round, making compost that's even better than that from an outdoor heap. Worms add their castings to the compost and make a dark and rich soil, and their LIFE CREATES a nutrifying fertilizer called "worm tea", used as a fast-acting soil supplement (MORE

PLEASE). Many people balk at the thought of having a box full of wriggling bait in their living rooms, but it's very easy to make their lair quite inconspicuous, and the slightly earthy and rich smell they create is pleasant to some and non-offensive to most.

> "From food all beings are born,
>
> By food they live and into food they return."
>
> - Taiitiriya Upanishad 3.2

Choosing a Worm Bin

The first thing you'll need to think about is size. Estimate the weight of a week's worth of food scraps, and plan on 1 square foot of surface area for every pound. A 2' x 4' box, for example, is large enough for eight pounds of kitchen scraps a week. The container will need to be 8 to 12 inches deep. A few small bins will be lighter and might be more manageable than one large one, but you'll have to feed the worms new kitchen scraps every few days so make sure not to have more bins than you can support.

Commercial bins are available in wood or plastic. Plastic tends to hold too much moisture, and while wood "breathes" and maintains the proper humidity, it is subject to rot and termites. Also, treated wood is toxic to worms, and many "found" wooden containers, which we'll discuss next, have questionable finishes. The best solution is to use redwood, hemlock, or untreated pine finished with 2 coats of non-toxic varnish. Wood is also a great insulator and will help to keep your bin the proper temperature, above freezing and below 80° Fahrenheit.

Buying 2 plastic totes, one inside of the other and one of

the lids underneath to protect the floor, is an easy and inexpensive solution. Discarded barrels, dresser drawers, or trunks work great too, and are not only free, they can also have way more personality that garish plastic totes or minimalist commercial worm bins. In fact, an entire dresser is an awesome worm bin with its multiple boxes (aka drawers) which are already covered by the drawers above. Holes are drilled through each drawer except the bottom one, which isn't filled with worms and dirt, but covered in plastic sheeting or painter's drop cloths to catch the worm tea. It looks like furniture (on account of that it is) and your guests don't need to know the slithery secret therein. Depending on the size of the dresser, the drawers can become quite heavy so look for a good sliding mechanism. Also, it's not a bad idea to put your worm bin on wheels or casters before you start.

You can also have a main bin outside or in a basement (great because it's warm, dark, and dry) and a mini-bin conveniently placed right in the kitchen, dumping the too-foody contents into a bigger bin and scooping a few inches of new dirt and dirt-makers before it's taken back to the kitchen counter.

Preparing your bin

Whatever container you choose, it must have adequate ventilation and drainage. Drill a few ¼" holes per square foot in the bottom to allow air to circulate in the underside of the biomass, and to allow drainage of the tea. If the material becomes too wet, drill some more holes up from the bottom. Put the bin on bricks or wooden blocks to allow air in, and put something underneath it, like a large tray or a plastic sheet with the edges laying over something to raise them up. The sides can then be gathered like a Santa Claus bag to remove the liquid fertilizer. The container needs a cover to keep out light and conserve moisture. If your bin is indoors, the darkness and seal provided by sliding a drawer in or closing the lid of a trunk is ideal. Otherwise, a piece of burlap thrown over the top is fine. An old coffee bean bag will make the worms very happy, and add a nice coffee smell to your earthy loam. If your bin is outside it's best to seal it up in such a way as to keep out pests and rain – but remember that worms are animals and need to breathe, so make sure your bin has adequate ventilation.

The bedding materials are the same for worms as for compost (see pg XX) with one exception – a couple of handfuls of sand or dirt will provide the grit worms' digestive tracks need. Add your brown matter and wet it to the consistency of a wrung-out sponge. It should form a ball when packed in the hand. Your bin is ready for worms and scraps.

Acquiring worms

The two types of worms best suited to vermiculture are both of the red variety: red wigglers (*Eisenia foetida),* and the less common *Lumbricus rubella.* They are found in aged manure and compost heaps. The cheapest route (and best story) is to go to a horse stable or farm and get permission to harvest them from some manure. Another way to gather redworms is to put a large piece of wet cardboard on your lawn, garden, or local park at night. The most virile worms will crawl upwards to feast on the wet cardboard. Lift up the cardboard in the morning to gather the your new co-gardeners. They can also be purchased from bait stores (but be careful of the species you're getting! Red wigglers are also called manure worm, red hybrid, striped worm, and fish worm, but night crawlers et al will not work) and online. Two pounds of worms can handle a pound of kitchen scraps daily, or a four square foot container. Worms can be pretty expensive at $20 per pound (about 1000 worms) but they will quickly multiply. Breeding worms can lay two or three cocoons per week which will hatch in 21 days, each cocoon producing two or three worms that will mature in 60 to 90 days. A worm population eventually stabilizes at a level that can be supported by the amount of food and space. If you're starting with a small Mayflower of pioneering wrigglers, start them slowly on small snacks until they're populous enough to decimate a (vegetarian) Thanksgiving dinner.

Care and feeding

Every meal to every few days, dig a little bit into the bedding material, bury your scraps and cover it over. Try to use a different spot each time to distribute the food evenly. Worms especially like melons, lettuce, and apples but you can feed them any vegetarian scraps, like fruit cores, rinds and peels, vegetable scraps, grains, or bread. Coffee grounds are much beloved, as well as the filters. Try to give them a variety of foods, and only a little bit of citrus so that the pH stays fairly neutral. The smaller you cut up your food scraps the faster they'll disappear, so high-speed blender and food processor waste is great. Make sure to cover the pits and peels with an inch or two of bedding; if you leave wet green matter uncovered it may attract fruit flies or smelly yeasts and molds. Otherwise, if you have a good ratio of worms to food scraps to area, your bin will manage itself for the 2 – 6 months it will take for the brown bedding material and all of the food scraps to be converted into chocolate-colored, homogeneous and glowingly fertile earth. This material is called "worm castings", and my favorite worm species, the "dirt pooper", sums up the process nicely. The end result will have majorly reduced in bulk, as the elemental particles have settled and compressed. It's important to be aware of this moment (which shouldn't be hard, as you're in there at least every few days, right?) as the worms will begin to die with nothing left to eat. They need to be separated from the castings and given a new home, and though there are complicated contraptions in commercial worm bins that let the soil fall out the bottom sans worms, there's a simpler way. Push all of the new soil to one side of the bin, and put a new batch of bedding in the open space. It's a great time to alter the bedding material, as different raw materials equals different nutrients, both for your worms and you plants. Start putting your food scraps in the new bedding and in a couple of weeks, the worms will flock to the new bedding like gay high-schoolers to traveling Broadway auditions. The soil can then be diluted to 1 part worm castings to 2-3 parts regular soil and used in your wheatgrass trays or to replace settled dirt in your container (the same settling has happened there as in the worm bin), saved in plastic bags, or just stored right there indefinitely. For container gardening, including grasses and micro greens, use. If you put your used soil in the bin with this end ratio in mind, you'll save yourself one more step. Full strength castings can be directly to the soil as a top fertilizer in pre-existing container plants.

If you want the fresh dirt immediately, want to check out the number of your worms, or want a fun project for the kids, you can just turn the bin over onto a garbage bag and remove the worms by hand. Watch for the lemon-shaped worm cocoons (or "capsules") that contain between 2 and 20 babies. They're actually much tougher than the worms themselves, but worth their weight in gold and easy to miss.

I leave you with two thoughts on either end of the spectrum. One deals with poop. The wasted manure and compost of your community: your police horses' droppings, your fields of cow pies, your neighbors' pet's poop tentatively scooped and sequestered into the illusion of sanitary little plastic bags. I guarantee that most of the best waste in your neighborhood is going to waste. I'm not suggesting you pick through piles of manure you find in fields (though one of our presidents didn't think it beneath him; in fact he found more joy in that endeavor than most others *see quote below) though I'll applaud you if you do, but what's to stop you from supplying your neighbors with a lidded bucket and a promise of weekly collection? Or setting up a "soil from soil" station at the local dog park? Just keeping those neatly tied sacs of droppings out of landfills is enough of a reason; the local gardeners that will clamor for the sweetly fragrant soil that you've carefully composted outdoors, and the boxes of free veggies *that* will bring, is just a bonus.

The other is a kind of prayer, the poetic offers of two guys passionate about earth. Not "the Earth", that vague and vast network of systems, each with its own politics and dogma, but *earth*, the actual stuff that land-dwelling animals daily quantify between their toes as home in the universe. These men were, I hope, far ahead of their time and not eulogizing the single force that creates, sustains, and destroys, building the very bodies of newborn babies from the rotting death of the millennia.

"In making experiments upon the varieties of Soils and Manures... you will find as much employment for your interest and as high a gratification to your good taste as in any business of amusement you wish to pursue. The finest productions of the Poet or Painter, the Statuary or the Architect, when they stand in competition with the great and beautiful operations of Nature, must be pronounced mean and despicable baubles." - John Adams, 2nd President of the US

and

"Behold this compost! behold it well!

Perhaps every mite has once form'd part of a sick person—
Yet behold!

The grass of spring covers the prairies,

The bean bursts noiselessly through the mould in the garden,

...

The summer growth is innocent and disdainful above all those strata of sour dead.

...

Now I am terrified at the Earth! it is that calm and patient,

It grows such sweet things out of such corruptions,

It turns harmless and stainless on its axis, with such endless successions of diseas'd corpses,

It distils such exquisite winds out of such infused fetor,

It renews with such unwitting looks, its prodigal, annual, sumptuous crops,

It gives such divine materials to men, and accepts such leavings from them at last.

Walt Whitman – from "This Compost". When our world finally celebrates its worms and nematodes and soil bacteria, this will be their anthem.

Appendix A - Plant Nutritional Deficiencies

Macronutrients

Calcium (Ca)

- **Symptoms:** New leaves are deformed or hook-shaped. The growing tip of a leaf turns brown and dies. Contributes to blossom end rot in tomatoes, tip burn of cabbage and internal browning in plants like escarole and celery.
- **Remedy:** Crushed eggshells sown about 2" down, Lime, or Gypsum (which should be used only in alkaline soils).
- **Notes:** Too much Ca will inhibit other nutrients, and is often a "transpiration" issue, that is, the plant is exhibiting the symptoms of a Ca deficiency not because of a shortage in the soil but because its roots can't breathe either from root-lock or too much moisture in the soil.

Nitrogen (N)

- **Symptoms:** Older leaves, generally at the bottom of the plant, will yellow. Remaining foliage is often light green. Stems may also yellow and may become spindly. Slow growth.
- **Remedy:** Manure is very rich in nitrogen, and can be sown directly into soil. Earthworm castings are wonderful, as are coffee grounds (acidic, add to alkaline soils only).
- **Notes:** Nitrogen is hugely important to plants, kind of like protein is important to weightlifters. Growing plants build themselves out of it, all the way down to their DNA. Be vigilant, because many forms of nitrogen are water soluble and wash away.

Magnesium (Mg)

- **Symptoms:** Slow growth and leaves turn pale yellow, sometimes just on the outer edges. New growth may be yellow with dark spots.
- **Remedy:** Compost, or Mix 1-2 teaspoons of Epsom salts per gallon of water until condition improves.
- **Notes:** Needed for photosynthesis, as the magnesium atom is central in the chlorophyll molecule. All plants can be deficient in magnesium, but tomato plants and apple trees are particularly prone.

Phosphorus (P)

- **Symptoms:** Small leaves that may take on a reddish-purple tint. Leaf tips can look burnt and older leaves become almost black. Reduced fruit or seed production.
- **Remedy:** Chicken manure (no need to compost it, just put it right in the soil), rock phosphate, ground-up bones (if you have any handy) or bonemeal.
- **Notes:** If your soil pH is above 7.3 or below 5, there may be plenty of phosphorous but it's been fixed and the plant can use it. Consider a pH amendment instead. Phosphorous must be mixed with water to be usable, so dissolve it first or water heavily after applying.

Potassium (K)

- **Symptoms:** Older leaves may look scorched around the edges and/or wilted. Interveinal chlorosis (yellowing between the leaf veins) develops.
- **Remedy:** Wood ash, which raises pH; potash magnesia is usually sold as "sul-po-mag", which also contains magnesium and sulfur, often absent alongside missing K.

    Notes: Needed for strong stems and disease resistance.

Sulfur (S)

- **Symptoms:** New growth is stunted and/or turns pale yellow while older growth stays green.
- **Remedy:** Mix 1-2 teaspoons of Epsom salts per gallon of water until condition improves.
- **Notes:** Sulfur plays an important role in root growth, chlorophyll supply and plant proteins. Just like iron, S moves slowly in the plant, and hotter temperatures will make S harder to absorb like iron. But unlike iron, S is distributed evenly throughout the plant which is why both new and old leaves are affected.

Micronutrients

Boron (B)

- **Symptoms:** Poor stem and root growth. Terminal (end) buds may die and immature flowers may fall off. Resembles Calcium deficiency (see Notes)
- **Remedy:** Treat with one teaspoon of Boric acid (sold as eyewash) per gallon of water. Can be applied as a foliar spray (directly to the leaves).
- **Notes:** Aids in cell division and protein formation, important in keeping calcium soluble and available to the plant. The most common deficiency in non-organic, over-worked soils; is a problem organic gardeners rarely encounter. Lucky us.

Copper (Cu)

- **Symptoms:** Stunted growth. Leaves can become limp, curl, or drop, and their tips can become blueish-green. Stalks can become limp and bend over.
- **Remedy:** Copper chelate, at about ¼ of the recommended rate
- **Notes:** Cu is influenced by soil pH and organic matter. Copper is unavailable above a pH of 7.5; peaty and acidic soils are most likely to be deficient. Unfinished compost can make copper unavailable in the soil.

Iron (Fe)

Symptoms: Young yellow leaves with green veins, symptoms which are often confused with nitrogen deficiency.

Remedy: Compost is best and quickest. Adding sulfur to the soil, which will turn into sulfuric acid and lower the pH, will make the existing iron more available. This will take a while.

Notes: Essential for plants to make chlorophyll, plays a role in the synthesis of plant proteins, and helps plants fix nitrogen. Fe deficiency is usually the result of too alkaline soils; at a pH above 6.8 Fe is fixed in the soil. Can also be caused by too much manganese…

Manganese (Mn)

- **Symptoms:** Growth slows. Younger leaves turn mottled, or spotted, yellow, often starting between veins. Veins may stay green. May develop dark or dead spots. Leaves, shoots and fruit diminished in size. Failure to bloom.
- **Remedy:** A handful of dolomitic limestone per gallon of soil.
- **Notes:** Helps enzymes break down for chlorophyll and photosynthesis production, as well as it works with plant enzymes to reduce nitrates before producing proteins.

Molybdenum (Mo)

- **Symptoms:** Older leaves yellow, remaining foliage turns light green. Leaves can become narrow and distorted.
- **Remedy:** Dolomitic limestone provides a tiny amount of Mo, but is effective in raising the soil pH, which is most likely the problem.**Notes:** A very rare deficiency. Acts as an enzyme co-factor to metabolize nitrogen they take up from the soil, so is often confused with nitrogen deficiency.

Zinc (Zn)

- **Symptoms:** Yellowing between veins of new growth. Terminal (end) leaves may form a rosette.
- **Remedy:** Manure, which decomposes quickly. Leaves and stems often fail to grow to normal size.
- **Notes:** Though a rare deficiency in organic plants, corn, potatoes and bean are the most susceptible.

Recommended Reading

Fermentation:

The Art of Fermentation: An In-Depth Exploration of Essential Concepts and Processes from Around the World by Sandor Ellix Katz and Michael Pollan

Wild Fermentation by Sandor Ellix Katz *with an incredible recommended reading list

Understanding: Bacteria Discovery Education School (DVD, and on youtube)

Sprouting:

Sprouts: The Miracle Food: The Complete Guide to Sprouting by Steve Meyerowitz and Michael Parman

The Sprouting Book: How to Grow and Use Sprouts to Maximize Your Health and Vitality by Ann Wigmore

The Wheatgrass Book: How to Grow and Use Wheatgrass to Maximize Your Health and Vitality by Ann Wigmore

Gardening:

Fresh Food from Small Spaces: The Square-Inch Gardener's Guide to Year-Round Growing, Fermenting, and Sprouting by R.J. Ruppenthal

Dirt: the Ecstatic Skin of the Earth by William Bryant Logan

Vegetarianism, Veganism, and Raw Food Prep:

Eating Animals by Jonathan Safran-Foer.

Diet for a New America and The Food Revolution by John Robbins.

Beyond Beef: The Rise and fall of the Cattle Culture by Jeremy Rifkin

RAW by Charlie Trotter

Ani's Raw Food Kitchen: Easy, Delectable Living Foods Recipes by Ani Phyo

Environment, GMOs, and Agribusiness:

The Power of Community: How Cuba Survived Peak Oil (DVD and on youtube)

The Weather of the Future by Heidi Cullen

Stolen Harvest: The Hijacking of the Global Food Supply by Dr. Vandana Shiva

The World According to Monsanto (DVD)

Evolution and Pleasure

Stumbling on Happiness by Daniel Gilbert

How Pleasure Works by Paul Bloom

Supernormal Stimuli: How Primal Urges Overran Their Evolutionary Purpose by Deidre Barrett

Resources:

Seeds, Grains and Nuts:

NutsOnline.com - A family business with great prices, customer service, and a touch of whimsy in everything they do. They once sent a stuffed elephant with my order. Sold.

Wheatgrasskits.com - A great source for certain seeds as well as sprouting supplies

Nutiva - The best hemp seeds and coconut oil. I get the 3-lb bag of organic shelled hempseeds and double pack of 54-oz jars of organic coconut oil, and I buy them through amazon.com to get free shipping and a "Subscribe and Save" discount. They also make a raw coconut oil which comes in glass and is great, and more expensive.

Sprouting Bags – available from great companies like Pure Joy Planet, but I use reusable mesh produce bags that are about 20 times cheaper and might last longer, but have a slightly wider mesh so the tiniest seeds like amaranth need the real deal. Or panty hose.

Probiotic Cultures

Dairy Kefir - kefirlady.com – a great source for dairy kefir grains grown in organic raw goat milk, and at the time of this writing she sells a ¼ cup for $20 with shipping; top-quality grains at the best price on the net for the quantity. Is also very available to answer questions and share the enthusiasm.

Kombucha, Juice Kefir, Apple Cider Vinegar – try your local craigslist first, then ebay. Can also be started from a raw and unflavored product from your local natural foods store.

Index

"The Worst Mistake in the History of the Human Race", 50
"open air" compost bin, 164
alfalfa, 59
algae, 120, 122, 158
alkalinity, 68, 82
Alkalinity, 68
allergies, 10
Alzheimer's, 70
amino acids, 15, 17, 61

ammonium nitrate, 37
Anheuser-Busch, 31
Ann Wigmore, 65, 182
antioxidants, 70
arthritis, 71
artificial light, 86
athlete's foot, 69
B1, 18
B12, 66, 71
bacteria, 21, 24, 25, 61, 62
basal ganglia, 55
bedding materials for worms, 171
beef, 35
blood pressure, 68
body odor, 69
brain, 21, 54, 55, 57
Brain, 53
bread, 59
burns, 69
Bush administration, 47
butter, 11, 13
cadmium, 68
Calcium, 17
cancer, 19, 23, 30, 50, 65, 71, 92
Cancer, 11
candida, 71
cars, 37, 39
Charile Bell, 50
cheese, 61
children, 23, 25, 40, 50, 51, 52, 53
China, 8, 29, 34, 39
chlorophyll, 64, 67, 70, 71, 86, 88, 106, 178, 179, 180
cholesterol, 51
cleansing, 73
colitis, 68
colon cancer, 50
composting, 159, 161, 164, 169
corn, 21, 24, 50, 52
Cuba, 39, 40, 41, 42, 43, 44
Dead Sea Scrolls, 64
diabetes, 44, 50
diarrhea, 68
dirt, 63, 76, 77, 78, 81, 82, 83, 84, 85, 86, 95, 97, 99, 100, 101, 103, 106, 108, 114, 117, 118, 144, 146, 155, 158, 159, 161, 170, 171, 173, 174, 182
DNA, 21, 22, 24, 47
Dr. Alexis Carrel, 73
Dr. Bernard Jensen, 70
Dr. Jared Diamond, 50
Dr. Rajendra Pachauri, 47
Dr. Watson, 47
Dr. Yoshihide Hagiwara, 65, 67
drug-addicted brain, 55
drugs, 29, 56
earthworm castings, 77
Easter Island, 45
Edmond Bordeaux Szekely, 64
effects of artificial light on pumpkins, 87
effects of different kinds of light on animals, 87
Eisenia foetida, 172

embargo of Cuba, 40
enzyme, 15, 50, 68, 70, 181
Enzyme Inhibitors, 15, 16
enzymes, 13, 15, 60, 61, 67, 68, 69, 72, 180
Enzymes, 60
Essene Gospels of Peace, 64
Eubie Blake, 74
evolution, 57
Exxon, 47
fast food, 8, 49, 52
fermented, 11
fertility, 70
fertilizer, 21, 29, 31, 37, 41, 42, 78, 83, 89, 90, 91, 97, 109, 119, 120, 158, 169, 171, 174
fiber, 15, 42
flax, 9
forest, 14, 22, 45, 46, 159, 161
free radicals, 60, 70
gas, 20, 38, 41, 43
Genetic Modification, 21
Germany, 57
ghee, 11
GMO, 21, 22, 24, 26, 28
GMO labelling, 10, 21, 28
goat milk, 13, 184
GOP, 44
grapefruit seed extract, 123
gray hair, 69
growing medium, 63, 64, 78, 85, 90, 94, 99, 100, 101, 103, 122, 127, 129, 130, 133, 134, 140, 141, 144, 145, 146, 150, 158
halitosis, 70
heart disease, 44, 50, 51
heavy metals, 70, 159
hemoglobin, 67
high blood pressure, 51
Hippocrates, 65
hormones, 51
hunter-gathererers, 49
hydrogen peroxide, 91
Hyper-Maturation, 49
immune system, 13
inductively coupled plasma spectometer, 76
infant mortality, 43
iron, 67, 70, 71, 179, 180
Iron, 18
John Ott, 86
Johns Hopkins University, 54
Kamut, 13
kefir, 11, 13, 184
Kid's menus, 51
kombucha, 12
lactation, 70
lactose, 10
lactose intolerance, 10
life expectancy, 43
lifespan, 50
light, 34, 76, 84, 86, 87, 88, 91, 94, 95, 98, 103, 104, 105, 106, 107, 109, 111, 117, 122, 123, 125, 142, 171, 177, 181

lipase, 11
liver, 68, 73, 113
Living foods, 59
Lumbricus rubella, 172
lust, 55
magnesium, 67, 72, 178
manure, 41, 77, 91, 162, 172, 174, 178
McDonald's, 49, 50, 53
McDonalds, 50
mercury, 27, 68
micro lettuces, 63, 97, 99
milk, 11, 13, 34, 50, 51
miso, 61
mold, 77, 78, 84, 85, 111
Monsanto, 22, 24, 26, 27, 31
Mung Beans, 17
mustard, 21
Myriad Genetics, 30
negative ions, 69
nerve cells, 54, 55
Nestle, 33
nicotine, 68
nitrogen, 17, 19, 21
Nobel Prize, 73
NPK, 19, 21
nut butter, 13
obesity, 51, 52, 68
Obesity, 51
Oil, 38
overweight children, 51
oxygen, 67, 69, 71, 92, 93, 94, 111, 115, 120, 122, 161, 163
Paleolithic, 49
passive composting, 164
Peak Oil, 37, 39

peas, 13, 34
peptic ulcers, 68
permaculture, 160
pesticide, 19, 22, 29
pesticides, 19, 21, 22, 23, 24, 31, 34, 37, 38, 41, 42
Peter Fitzgerald, 52
phosphorous, 19
pleasure, 9, 57
poison ivy, 69
polyvinyl chloride, 69
poop, 174
potassium, 19
Potassium, 18
pre-frontal cortex, 55
protein, 17, 21, 61
PSRAST, 25
pumpkin, 9
QAI, 34
recycling, 91, 113, 122
red wigglers, 172
rice, 34, 50, 52
sagging skin, 68
salt, 49, 50
saturated fats, 51
sauerkraut, 13
Seed/Nut Digestibility Chart, 60
sexual maturity, 51
shoots, 97, 100
sleep, 69, 74, 160
SOD, 70
sodium, 18
soil, 19, 20, 22, 29, 41, 42, 45, 63, 64, 77, 78, 79, 80, 81, 82, 83, 89, 90, 92, 97, 99, 103,

106, 107, 108, 109,
111, 112, 113, 114,
115, 116, 117, 118,
129, 134, 146, 150,
159, 160, 161, 162,
163, 169, 173, 174,
176, 177, 178, 180, 181
soilless media, 82
Soviet Union, 40, 43
starch, fat, and salt, 49
sterilizing soil, 78
Steve Meyerowitz, 64,
182
strokes, 44
strontium, 68
sugar, 52
Sugar mills, 43
sunflower lettuce, 101
sunlight, 86, 127
Taiitiriya Upanishad, 169
Target, 34
terminator gene, 26
TerraChoice, 33
The Future of Food, 26
thyroid, 68
Time Lapse Research
   Laboratory, 87
topsoil, 29, 46
trans-fats, 51
travelling, 19

tryptophan, 24, 25
tumors, 68, 69
ulcers, 69
United Nations
   Intergovernmental
   Panel on Climate
   Change, 47
USDA, 31
vegan diet, 67
vermiculture, 161, 169,
   172
Wal-mart, 31
water, 15, 29, 33, 43, 60,
   61
water heaters, 43
Wendy's, 33
wheat, 13, 50
wheatgrass, 64, 66, 67,
   68, 70, 182
WHO. *See* World Health
   Organization
Whole Foods, 13, 34
Willpower, 54
World Health
   Organization, 52
worms, 41, 159, 162, 169,
   170, 171, 172, 173,
   174, 176
yoga, 9, 49

Stay Connected!

Visit

www.KitchenSinkFarming.org

for tips, recipes, news, giveaways, and general delicious nerdiness.